BEYOND TREMORS:

The Unexpected Tools You Need To Thrive With Parkinson's Disease

By

Linda J. Scott.

TABLE OF CONTENTS

CHAPTER 3: Building Your Wellness Arsenal: Traditional Therapies

CHAPTER 4: Beyond Medications: Exploring Complementary and Alternative Therapies

CHAPTER 5: The Power of Your Network: Navigating Support Systems

CHAPTER 6: Living Well, Not Just Managing: Redefining Your Quality of Life

CHAPTER 7: Advocating for Yourself: Taking Charge of Your Healthcare

CHAPTER 8: Looking Ahead: The Future of Parkinson's Research and Treatment

CHAPTER 9: A Final Note: Living Beyond Limitations

INTRODUCTION

Welcome, dear reader, to a journey that goes beyond the tremors, beyond the diagnosis, and into the heart of resilience and empowerment in the face of Parkinson's disease. As we embark on this exploration together, I invite you to leave preconceptions at the door and open your mind to the unexpected tools and possibilities that await.

In these pages, we won't merely discuss Parkinson's; we'll engage in a conversation about living well, thriving, and finding strength in the face of challenges. This is not just a book; it's a guide, a companion, and a source of inspiration for individuals navigating the landscape of Parkinson's and those supporting them.

As someone who has walked the path of Parkinson's, I understand the fears, uncertainties, and questions that may accompany this journey. My goal is to shift the narrative away from the sole focus on tremors and dive into the myriad aspects of Parkinson's – from the physical to the emotional, from the myths to the realities.

Together, we'll explore traditional and complementary therapies, build a robust support network, and delve into the promising future of Parkinson's research and treatment. This is a conversation about living beyond limitations, setting realistic goals, and celebrating the victories, big and small.

Whether you're someone living with Parkinson's, a caregiver, or a healthcare professional, I invite you to join me in this exploration. Let's navigate the unexpected and empower each other to embrace a life that extends far beyond the diagnosis.

Onward to a journey of understanding, support, and the unwavering belief that life with Parkinson's can be not just manageable but truly fulfilling.

CHAPTER 1

Beyond the Tremors: Unveiling the Many Faces of Parkinson's

Shifting the Narrative Away from Tremors as the Sole Focus

Hey there,

I'm thrilled to embark on this journey with you in exploring life beyond Parkinson's disease. I know firsthand the challenges that come with this condition, and it's my aim to share insights that go beyond the commonly spotlighted aspect: tremors.

Picture this – Parkinson's is often painted as a one-dimensional story, dominated by the visible tremors that characterize the condition. However, in this book, we're about to flip that narrative. It's time to broaden our perspective and delve into the multifaceted nature of Parkinson's.

As someone who has navigated the twists and turns of Parkinson's, I've come to realize that focusing solely on tremors can overshadow the myriad other aspects that define this journey. This book is not just about understanding the science behind Parkinson's; it's about recognizing the full spectrum of symptoms – both the visible motor challenges and the subtle, yet equally impactful, non-motor aspects.

In the pages that follow, we'll venture into the intricate web of Parkinson's, unraveling the myths, exploring various tools for well-being, and most importantly, shining a light on the often-overlooked elements that can empower you to not just cope but truly thrive.

So, buckle up for a ride that transcends the expected. We're about to discover tools, strategies, and perspectives that will redefine what it means to live with Parkinson's. I invite you to join me in this exploration, where we'll not only address the challenges but also uncover unexpected avenues for a fulfilling life.

Let's shift the narrative, broaden our understanding, and embark on a journey that goes Beyond Tremors.

Understanding Parkinson's: Breaking Down the Science in an Accessible Way

Let's dive into the heart of the matter: Parkinson's disease. It's a topic that can seem daunting at first glance, but fear not – I'm here to break it down in a way that's easy to grasp.

At its core, Parkinson's is a neurological disorder that affects movement. It's named after Dr. James Parkinson, who first described the condition in 1817. Essentially, Parkinson's occurs when certain nerve cells in the brain, particularly those producing dopamine, become damaged or die off. Now, dopamine is a crucial neurotransmitter responsible for transmitting signals that coordinate movement. So, when these dopamine-producing cells start to falter, it disrupts the brain's ability to regulate movement smoothly.

You might wonder, "What causes this damage to occur?" Well, that's where things get a bit tricky. Parkinson's is considered a multifactorial condition, meaning it's influenced by a combination of genetic, environmental, and possibly even lifestyle factors. While researchers have identified certain genetic mutations associated with Parkinson's, the majority of cases are believed to be sporadic, with no clear genetic link.

Now, let's talk about the hallmark symptoms of Parkinson's. Most people are familiar with the motor symptoms, such as tremors, rigidity, bradykinesia (slowness of movement), and postural instability. These are often the telltale signs that lead to a diagnosis. However, Parkinson's is more than just a movement disorder – it can also manifest with a wide range of non-motor symptoms. These can include cognitive changes, mood disorders, sleep disturbances, and even gastrointestinal issues.

Diagnosing Parkinson's isn't always straightforward. It typically involves a thorough medical history, a comprehensive physical examination, and sometimes additional tests, such as brain imaging or specialized movement assessments. Early signs of Parkinson's can be subtle and easily overlooked, which is why it's important to seek medical attention if you notice any concerning symptoms.

So, in a nutshell, Parkinson's is a complex neurological condition characterized by a disruption in the brain's ability to control movement, stemming from the loss of dopamine-producing cells. While the exact cause remains elusive, researchers continue to unravel the mysteries of Parkinson's in hopes of developing more effective treatments and ultimately, finding a cure.

UNDERSTANDING THE DIFFERENT STAGES OF PARKINSON'S DISEASE

Parkinson's disease (PD) manifests uniquely in each individual. Not all symptoms may present themselves, and if they do, the order and intensity can vary greatly.

Understanding the typical stages of Parkinson's can provide valuable guidance for navigating its progression. While some individuals may experience these stages over the course of two decades or more, others might see a faster advancement of the disease.

Predicting the trajectory of Parkinson's progression is challenging. Following diagnosis, many individuals respond well to medications like levodopa. This positive response can span several years, but the duration differs for each person.

Yet, as Parkinson's advances, adjustments to levodopa dosages often become necessary, requiring collaboration between the individual and their healthcare provider. During this phase, new or worsening movement symptoms may arise, including levodopa-induced dyskinesia, swallowing difficulties, gait freezing, falls, and balance issues.

Those diagnosed with young-onset PD are at a higher risk of levodopa-induced dyskinesia and motor fluctuations, while older individuals may encounter more cognitive changes and non-movement symptoms.

Motor fluctuations typically arise five to ten years post-diagnosis, while postural instability, leading to balance issues and falls, tends to manifest after around a decade.

Stages	Explanation
1	In the early stages of Parkinson's, individuals typically experience mild symptoms that don't significantly disrupt their daily activities. Tremors and other movement-related symptoms tend to manifest on one side of the body. Additionally, changes in posture, walking, and facial expressions become noticeable during this phase. These symptoms may be subtle, allowing the person to continue with their regular

		routines without significant interference.
2		As the disease progresses, symptoms intensify. Tremors, rigidity, and other movement-related issues begin to impact both sides of the body or extend to the midline, affecting areas like the neck and trunk. Walking problems and noticeable posture issues may become more apparent. Despite the challenges, individuals in this stage can still live independently, although daily tasks become more arduous and time-consuming. The increased difficulty in performing routine activities marks a shift in the impact of Parkinson's on daily life.
3		Entering the mid-stage, a defining characteristic is the loss of balance, evident in unsteadiness during turns or when the individual is pushed while standing, leading to a higher risk of falls. Motor symptoms persist and worsen during this phase. Functionally, there is a noticeable restriction in daily activities, yet the person remains physically capable of maintaining an independent lifestyle. Disability, at this stage, is generally mild to moderate, reflecting the evolving impact of Parkinson's on daily functioning.
4		In this advanced stage, symptoms are fully

	developed and profoundly disabling. While the individual may still have the ability to walk and stand independently, there's a heightened need for safety, often requiring the use of a cane or walker. Assistance with activities of daily living becomes crucial, and the person is no longer able to live independently. This phase signifies a significant shift in the level of support and care required due to the increased challenges posed by Parkinson's disease.
5	In the most advanced and debilitating stage, stiffness in the legs may reach a point where standing or walking becomes impossible. The individual is either bedridden or confined to a wheelchair, reliant on assistance for all activities. Around-the-clock care becomes a necessity, reflecting the profound impact of Parkinson's disease on the person's mobility and independence. This stage represents a challenging and demanding phase that requires continuous support and attention to address the comprehensive care needs of the individual.

Understanding the Origins of Parkinson's Disease: A Comprehensive Overview

When delving into the intricacies of Parkinson's disease, it becomes evident that various factors contribute to its onset. While some risk factors, like exposure to pesticides, are established, the primary causes remain elusive. Parkinson's is often categorized as "idiopathic," denoting a condition that seems to be a disease of its own, as scientists grapple with the challenge of pinpointing its precise origins.

Hereditary Influences: Familial Parkinson's Disease

Approximately 10% of Parkinson's cases are linked to a hereditary predisposition, where individuals inherit the condition from one or both parents. Researchers have identified seven distinct genes associated with Parkinson's, with three of them linked to early-onset forms of the disease. Certain genetic mutations contribute to unique traits, further complicating the understanding of this complex condition.

Unraveling the Mystery: Idiopathic Parkinson's Disease

The majority of Parkinson's cases fall under the category of idiopathic, suggesting that the cause is not inherited. Experts posit that this form of the disease arises from challenges in the body's processing of a protein called α-synuclein. When proteins undergo misfolding, assuming an incorrect shape, they accumulate in various regions or cells, forming Lewy bodies. Unlike hereditary forms, the presence of Lewy bodies in idiopathic cases triggers toxic effects and cell destruction.

Protein misfolding, a phenomenon not exclusive to Parkinson's, is observed in various diseases like Alzheimer's, Huntington's, and amyloidosis, highlighting the broader implications of this cellular dysfunction.

Parkinsonism and External Factors: Induced Parkinsonism

Distinct from authentic Parkinson's disease, induced parkinsonism shares similar traits but is triggered by external factors. Recognizing these causes is crucial for accurate diagnosis and appropriate treatment. Several factors linked to induced parkinsonism include:

- Drugs: Certain medications can induce Parkinsonism-like symptoms, which are usually reversible upon discontinuation. However, these effects may persist for weeks or even months after ceasing the medication.

- Encephalitis: Inflammation of the brain, known as encephalitis, can occasionally manifest as parkinsonism, underscoring the diverse ways in which neurological conditions can emerge.
- Toxins and Poisons: Exposure to various chemicals, such as manganese dust, carbon monoxide, welding fumes, or certain pesticides, has been associated with the development of parkinsonism.
- Injuries and Trauma: Repeated head injuries from high-impact sports like boxing, football, and hockey can result in brain damage, leading to a condition known as "post-traumatic parkinsonism."

Understanding these nuanced aspects of Parkinson's disease is crucial for both individuals affected by the condition and the medical community striving to advance treatments and interventions. The multifaceted nature of Parkinson's highlights the importance of ongoing research to unravel its complexities and pave the way for more targeted therapeutic approaches.

The Spectrum of Symptoms: Exploring Both Motor and Non-Motor Aspects

Now that we've dipped our toes into the science behind Parkinson's & also it's different stages, let's delve deeper into the rich tapestry of symptoms that define this complex condition. Parkinson's is like a multifaceted puzzle, with both motor and non-motor pieces contributing to the overall picture.

Firstly, the motor symptoms – the ones that often take center stage. You're probably familiar with the hallmark tremors, those rhythmic and involuntary movements that can affect different parts of the body. But Parkinson's has more tricks up its sleeve. Rigidity, or stiffness in the muscles, can make movement uncomfortable and challenging. Bradykinesia, or slowness of movement, can turn simple tasks into deliberate, effortful actions. Postural instability, another motor symptom, increases the risk of falls, adding another layer to the physical challenges.

Yet, Parkinson's isn't confined to its motor domain. There's a whole spectrum of non-motor symptoms that can be just as impactful, if not more so. Picture this: changes in cognition, such as difficulties with memory and attention, creating a cognitive landscape that demands adaptability. Mood swings and disorders, ranging from mild anxiety to more pronounced depression, can cast shadows over the emotional landscape. Sleep disturbances, like insomnia or restless legs, can turn nights into a restless battleground.

And then there are the less-discussed, yet equally significant, non-motor symptoms. Imagine grappling with gastrointestinal issues, like constipation, that silently contribute to the overall challenge. It's a reminder that Parkinson's is more than what meets the eye – it's a symphony of symptoms, each playing its unique role.

Navigating this spectrum requires a comprehensive approach. Medical professionals often assess the full range of symptoms to tailor treatment plans that address both motor and non-motor challenges. It's not just about managing visible tremors but also addressing the subtler, often underestimated, aspects that influence daily life.

SYMPTOMS AND CAUSES

What Are The Symptoms?

The most recognizable signs of Parkinson's disease involve the loss of muscular control. However, it's now understood that issues related to muscular control are not the sole potential indicators of Parkinson's disease.

Motor-related Symptoms:

Motor symptoms, implying movement-related issues, in Parkinson's disease include the following:

- Slowed Movements (Bradykinesia): A diagnosis of Parkinson's disease requires the manifestation of this symptom. Individuals experiencing it often interpret it as muscular weakness, though it arises from difficulties in muscle control rather than true strength loss.
- Tremor While Muscles Are at Rest: Approximately 80% of Parkinson's disease patients experience rhythmic muscle shaking even when not actively using those muscles. Resting tremors differ from essential tremors, which typically do not occur when muscles are at rest.
- Rigidity or Stiffness: Lead-pipe rigidity and cogwheel stiffness are common signs. Lead-pipe rigidity is a consistent, unchanging stiffness during movement, while cogwheel stiffness combines tremor with lead-pipe rigidity, resulting in jerky, stop-and-go motions, resembling the second hand of a mechanical clock.

- Unstable Posture or Walking Gait: Slower movements and rigidity in Parkinson's disease lead to a hunched-over or stooped posture, particularly as the condition worsens. This is evident in shorter, shuffling steps with reduced arm movement, and turning while walking may require more steps.

Additional Motor Symptoms Can Include:

- Blinking less frequently than normal, indicating diminished control of facial muscles.
- Cramped or tiny handwriting (micrographia) due to muscular control issues.
- Drooling, resulting from a lack of facial muscular control.
- Mask-like facial expression (hypomimia), with minimal or no alteration in facial expressions.
- Trouble swallowing (dysphagia) due to diminished throat muscular control, increasing the risk of issues like pneumonia or choking.
- Unusually quiet speaking voice (hypophonia) arising from diminished muscular control in the neck and chest.

Non-motor Symptoms:

Several symptoms unrelated to movement and muscle control are conceivable. Previously, specialists considered non-motor symptoms as potential risk factors when observed before motor symptoms. However, mounting evidence suggests these symptoms may appear in the early stages of the illness, potentially serving as warning indications years or even decades before motor difficulties.

Non-Motor Symptoms (with potential early warning symptoms in bold) Include:

- Autonomic Nervous System Symptoms, such as orthostatic hypotension (low blood pressure while standing up), constipation, gastrointestinal issues, urine incontinence, and sexual dysfunctions.
- Depression.
- Loss of sense of smell (anosmia).
- Sleep difficulties, including periodic limb movement disorder (PLMD), rapid eye movement (REM) behavior disorder, and restless legs syndrome.
- Trouble thinking and concentration (Parkinson's-related dementia).

Understanding this spectrum is key to living well with Parkinson's. It's about recognizing that every symptom, whether motor or non-motor, contributes to the unique journey each individual faces. And, more importantly, it's about embracing a holistic approach that goes beyond the visible tremors, acknowledging and addressing the entire spectrum of experiences.

As we continue this exploration, keep in mind that each symptom tells a part of your story with Parkinson's. By understanding and navigating this spectrum, you're not just managing the condition – you're navigating a unique and personal journey.

Diagnosis Journey: From Early Signs to Confirmation, Addressing Fears and Anxieties

Embarking on the diagnosis journey for Parkinson's is a process filled with twists, turns, and, undoubtedly, a rollercoaster of emotions. Let's navigate this path together, addressing not only the clinical aspects but also the very real fears and anxieties that often accompany it.

Early Signs: The Unspoken Whispers

You might begin to notice subtle changes – a slight tremor in your hand, a stiffness that wasn't there before, or perhaps a feeling of slowness in your movements. These whispers of change often signal the early stages of Parkinson's. It's essential to pay attention to these cues and, more importantly, to communicate them openly with your healthcare provider.

Seeking Answers: The Importance of Consultation
As you recognize these signs, the next step is seeking medical advice. This involves sharing your symptoms and concerns with a healthcare professional who can conduct a thorough examination. This process is not just about checking off a list of symptoms; it's about building a partnership with your healthcare team, ensuring that they understand your unique experience.

Addressing Fears and Anxieties: The Emotional Landscape
The road to a Parkinson's diagnosis can be emotionally charged. Fear of the unknown, anxiety about the future, and the weight of uncertainty can cast long shadows. It's perfectly normal to experience these emotions, and acknowledging them is a crucial step in the journey. Your healthcare provider is not just there to diagnose and treat; they are a valuable resource for addressing the emotional toll that comes with Parkinson's.

Confirming the Diagnosis: Navigating the Verdict

The moment of diagnosis can be a pivotal one. It's a confirmation of what you might have suspected, a label that can stir a mix of emotions. It's okay to feel a range of responses – relief at having an answer, uncertainty about what lies ahead, or even grief for the life you once knew. Your healthcare team plays a pivotal role during this stage, providing not just medical guidance but also emotional support.

Developing a Plan: The Path Forward

Following confirmation, the focus shifts to developing a comprehensive plan tailored to your unique needs. This involves discussing treatment options, lifestyle adjustments, and strategies for managing both motor and non-motor symptoms. The journey doesn't end with a diagnosis; it's a starting point for a collaborative effort between you and your healthcare team.

Support Systems: Building a Safety Net

Alongside medical professionals, building a robust support system is crucial. This includes family, friends, and, if needed, mental health professionals who can provide a safety net during moments of uncertainty. Joining Parkinson's support groups can connect you with individuals who share similar experiences, fostering a sense of community and understanding.

Remember, the diagnosis journey is not a solo expedition. It's a collective effort, involving healthcare professionals, loved ones, and, most importantly, you. By addressing fears and anxieties head-on, you're not just navigating the path to diagnosis – you're laying the foundation for a resilient journey with Parkinson's.

CHAPTER 2

Myths vs. Facts: Separating Truth from Fiction

Debunking Common Misconceptions about Parkinson's: Separating Fact from Fiction

Let's tackle head-on some of the most pervasive misconceptions surrounding Parkinson's disease. Dispelling these myths is not just about correcting information; it's about empowering you with accurate knowledge and fostering a deeper understanding of this complex condition.

MYTH: Parkinson's is just an "old person's disease."
FACT: While age is a significant risk factor, young-onset Parkinson's can affect individuals under 50. It's not exclusively an ailment of the elderly.

MYTH: Tremors are the only symptom of Parkinson's.

FACT: Parkinson's encompasses a broad range of symptoms, from motor challenges like tremors to non-motor aspects such as cognitive changes and mood disorders.

MYTH: Parkinson's is always hereditary.
FACT: While genetics can play a role, the majority of Parkinson's cases are sporadic, with no clear family link. It's a complex interplay of genetic and environmental factors.

MYTH: Only movement is affected; cognitive function remains intact.
FACT: Cognitive changes, including memory and attention issues, are common in Parkinson's and can significantly impact daily life.

MYTH: Parkinson's is contagious.
FACT: Parkinson's is not infectious. It's a neurodegenerative disorder influenced by a combination of genetic and environmental factors.

MYTH: If you have a tremor, it's definitely Parkinson's.
FACT: Tremors can have various causes, and not all tremors are indicative of Parkinson's. A thorough medical evaluation is crucial for an accurate diagnosis.

MYTH: Parkinson's is only about physical symptoms.

FACT: Non-motor symptoms, such as mood disorders and sleep disturbances, are integral components of Parkinson's and can impact overall well-being.

MYTH: Everyone with Parkinson's experiences the same symptoms.

FACT: Parkinson's is highly individualized, and symptoms can vary widely among individuals. What works for one person may not for another.

MYTH: Parkinson's medications stop the progression of the disease.

FACT: Medications can alleviate symptoms, but there is currently no cure for Parkinson's, and the disease progresses over time.

MYTH: Parkinson's is a normal part of aging.

FACT: While age is a risk factor, Parkinson's is not a normal part of aging. It's a distinct medical condition that requires proper diagnosis and management.

MYTH: People with Parkinson's can't lead fulfilling lives.

FACT: With the right support and management strategies, individuals with Parkinson's can lead active, fulfilling lives, pursuing their passions and goals.

MYTH: Parkinson's is only about physical challenges; it doesn't affect emotions.
FACT: Mood disorders, including anxiety and depression, are common in Parkinson's and need to be addressed alongside physical symptoms.

MYTH: Parkinson's is solely a movement disorder; it doesn't affect thinking.
FACT: Cognitive changes, often referred to as Parkinson's disease dementia, can occur as the condition progresses.

MYTH: Parkinson's is always visibly noticeable.
FACT: Some individuals with Parkinson's may not exhibit visible symptoms, especially in the early stages. Non-motor symptoms can be just as significant.

MYTH: If you don't have a family history, you won't get Parkinson's.
FACT: While family history can increase the risk, many individuals with Parkinson's have no family connection. Environmental factors also play a role.

MYTH: Parkinson's medications cause addictive behavior.

FACT: While impulse control disorders can occur as a side effect of certain medications, not everyone will experience these effects.

MYTH: People with Parkinson's are always in pain.

FACT: Pain is not a universal symptom of Parkinson's. While some individuals may experience pain, others may not.

MYTH: Parkinson's is a death sentence.

FACT: While Parkinson's is a chronic condition, it is not a direct cause of death. Many individuals live for decades with the condition.

MYTH: Only neurologists can diagnose Parkinson's.

FACT: While neurologists are often involved in the diagnosis, other healthcare professionals, such as movement disorder specialists, can also contribute to an accurate diagnosis.

MYTH: There's nothing you can do to slow the progression of Parkinson's.

FACT: While there is no cure, lifestyle factors like exercise and a healthy diet may help manage symptoms and improve overall well-being.

MYTH: Parkinson's can be cured through alternative therapies alone.

FACT: While complementary therapies may offer symptom relief, they are not a substitute for conventional medical treatments.

MYTH: People with Parkinson's should avoid physical activity.

FACT: Regular exercise is beneficial for individuals with Parkinson's, helping to improve mobility, balance, and overall quality of life.

MYTH: Parkinson's only affects movements; speech is not impacted.

FACT: Speech and communication can be affected by Parkinson's, leading to changes in voice volume and articulation.

MYTH: Parkinson's is the same for everyone; one-size-fits-all treatments work.

FACT: Personalized treatment plans are crucial, as individuals respond differently to medications and therapies.

MYTH: Parkinson's only affects men.

FACT: While men are slightly more likely to develop Parkinson's, it affects both men and women.

MYTH: Parkinson's is purely a brain disorder; it doesn't affect other organs.
FACT: Parkinson's can impact various organs, leading to non-motor symptoms such as gastrointestinal issues.

MYTH: Parkinson's can be prevented with a specific diet.
FACT: While a healthy diet is beneficial for overall well-being, there is no specific diet that can prevent Parkinson's.

MYTH: Deep Brain Stimulation (DBS) cures Parkinson's.
FACT: DBS can alleviate symptoms, but it is not a cure. Parkinson's remains a chronic condition.

MYTH: Parkinson's medications always cause side effects.
FACT: While medications can have side effects, not everyone will experience them, and adjustments can often be made to manage side effects.

MYTH: Parkinson's is purely a physical challenge; it doesn't affect cognition.

FACT: Cognitive changes are common in Parkinson's, and individuals may experience difficulties with memory, attention, and other cognitive functions.

MYTH: Parkinson's is only diagnosed in the later stages when tremors are prominent.
FACT: Early signs of Parkinson's can be subtle, and a diagnosis may occur before visible tremors develop.

MYTH: Parkinson's only affects white individuals.
FACT: Parkinson's can affect people of all racial and ethnic backgrounds.

MYTH: Parkinson's is an autoimmune disorder.
FACT: Parkinson's is not considered an autoimmune disorder; it is a neurodegenerative condition.

MYTH: Smoking prevents Parkinson's.
FACT: While some studies suggest a lower risk of Parkinson's in smokers, the health risks associated with smoking outweigh any potential protective effects.

MYTH: Parkinson's is always a rapidly progressing disease.

FACT: Parkinson's progression varies among individuals; some may experience slow progression, while others may progress more rapidly.

MYTH: Parkinson's only affects movement on one side of the body.
FACT: While symptoms often begin on one side, they can eventually affect both sides as the disease progresses.

MYTH: If you have a family member with Parkinson's, you'll definitely get it too.
FACT: While genetics can increase the risk, it does not guarantee that you will develop Parkinson's.

MYTH: Parkinson's is solely a result of head injuries.
FACT: While head injuries may contribute to the risk, the majority of Parkinson's cases have no history of significant head trauma.

MYTH: Parkinson's is a result of toxins in the environment alone.
FACT: Environmental factors can contribute to Parkinson's risk, but the interplay with genetic factors is complex.

MYTH: Parkinson's only affects the elderly; there's no need to worry about it at a younger age.

FACT: Young-onset Parkinson's can affect individuals under 50, emphasizing the importance of awareness and early detection.

Navigating Parkinson's requires accurate information. By debunking these myths, I aim to empower you with knowledge, fostering a clearer understanding of the challenges and possibilities that come with this condition.

Understanding Risk Factors: Genetics, Environment, and Lifestyle Influences

Let's unravel the intricate web of factors that contribute to the risk of Parkinson's disease. It's a mosaic influenced by genetics, environmental exposures, and lifestyle choices – a unique blend that shapes the likelihood of this complex condition.

Genetics: Unraveling the Inherited Threads

The role of genetics in Parkinson's is like examining a family album with a mix of familiar and mysterious faces. While some cases do have a hereditary component, with specific genetic mutations associated with Parkinson's, the majority are sporadic. In other words, you may not find a direct link in your family tree.

However, if you do have a family member with Parkinson's, it's worth paying attention. Certain genetic variations can indeed increase the risk, acting as potential markers in the genetic landscape. But remember, genetics alone don't dictate the entire story; they're just one piece of the puzzle.

Environment: Navigating External Influences
Imagine the environment as the backdrop of a play – it sets the stage for the unfolding narrative. In the context of Parkinson's, exposure to certain environmental factors can contribute to the risk. Pesticides, herbicides, and industrial chemicals are among the players that may influence the development of Parkinson's. Living or working in environments with increased exposure to these substances may add complexity to the risk landscape.

This doesn't mean you need to live in a bubble. Rather, it's about being aware and mindful of your surroundings. Awareness empowers you to make informed choices and, when possible, minimize potential exposures that may contribute to the risk.

Lifestyle: Nurturing Your Well-being

Your lifestyle choices are like the daily script you write for yourself – they shape the narrative of your health. Engaging in regular physical activity, maintaining a balanced diet, and prioritizing overall well-being can be powerful allies in mitigating the risk of Parkinson's.

Research suggests that individuals who engage in moderate to vigorous physical activity may have a lower risk of developing Parkinson's. Think of it as a pact with your body – by keeping it active and healthy, you're fostering resilience against potential challenges.

Nutrition plays a crucial role too. While no specific diet guarantees immunity, a diet rich in antioxidants, omega-3 fatty acids, and other neuroprotective elements may contribute to overall brain health. It's not about restrictive regimes but rather about nurturing your body with the fuel it needs to thrive.

And then there's the complex relationship with caffeine and nicotine. Studies hint at a potential protective effect, but the key lies in moderation. It's not an endorsement to take up smoking or downing excessive cups of coffee. Instead, it's a reminder that lifestyle choices, when made consciously and in moderation, can play a role in shaping your health narrative.

The Interplay: Your Unique Story
Now, picture all these factors interwoven, creating a tapestry that is uniquely yours. Your genetic makeup, the environment you navigate, and the choices you make – they all contribute to the canvas of your health.

Understanding risk factors is not about succumbing to fear but rather about informed empowerment. It's recognizing that your journey with Parkinson's is shaped by a combination of elements, each with its own influence. By gaining insights into these factors, you're not just a passive observer; you become an active participant in shaping your health narrative.

As we continue this exploration, keep in mind that knowledge is a compass guiding you through the complexities. By understanding the threads of genetics, the influences of your environment, and the impact of lifestyle choices, you're navigating your unique story with Parkinson's.

The Power of Early Intervention: Dispelling Myths about Delaying Diagnosis

Let's embark on a journey into the critical realm of early intervention in Parkinson's disease. There's a prevailing misconception that delaying a diagnosis is a benign choice, but in reality, early intervention can be a game-changer. Let's debunk the myths surrounding the timing of diagnosis and explore the profound impact of stepping into action sooner rather than later.

MYTH: "It's just a tremor – nothing to worry about."

One common misconception is downplaying the significance of early symptoms, such as a slight tremor or stiffness. The thought may be, "It's just part of aging," or "It's not affecting my daily life significantly." However, these early signs can be subtle precursors to Parkinson's. Acknowledging and addressing them promptly is not an overreaction; it's a proactive step towards understanding and managing the condition.

REALITY: Early diagnosis opens doors to timely management.

Contrary to the myth, an early diagnosis doesn't mean overmedicalization. Instead, it provides a window of opportunity for timely and targeted interventions. Early-stage Parkinson's allows healthcare professionals to implement strategies that can potentially slow down the progression of the disease and manage symptoms more effectively.

MYTH: "I don't want to burden my doctor with minor symptoms."

There's a tendency to downplay symptoms during medical visits, fearing they might not be significant enough to warrant attention. However, early symptoms may be indicative of underlying issues. Communicating openly with your healthcare provider is not a burden but an essential step towards an accurate diagnosis.

REALITY: Your doctor is a crucial ally in the early stages.

Healthcare providers are there to listen and evaluate. Sharing even minor symptoms allows them to piece together a comprehensive picture of your health. In the early stages of Parkinson's, these seemingly minor symptoms can be crucial clues. Your doctor becomes a partner in navigating the complexities of early intervention, guiding you towards the most appropriate strategies for your unique situation.

MYTH: "I'll wait until it gets worse to seek help."

Delaying seeking help often stems from a misconception that only significant impairment warrants attention. This myth assumes that intervention is only beneficial in advanced stages, but the opposite is true. Addressing symptoms early provides a foundation for better management and improved quality of life.

REALITY: Early intervention empowers you with choices.

In the realm of Parkinson's, knowledge truly is power. Early intervention allows you to explore a range of management options – from lifestyle adjustments and physical therapy to medication strategies. It's about giving you the agency to make informed choices and actively participate in shaping your journey with Parkinson's.

MYTH: "I'd rather not know; ignorance is bliss."

The fear of a Parkinson's diagnosis may lead some to adopt an "ignorance is bliss" approach. However, avoiding the truth doesn't alter the reality. Early knowledge is not a sentence but a catalyst for informed decision-making and proactive management.

REALITY: Knowledge is a powerful ally.

Understanding your health status empowers you to plan for the future, make lifestyle adjustments, and engage in interventions that can positively impact your well-being. Early knowledge enables you to approach Parkinson's not as an insurmountable challenge but as a condition to be managed with resilience and informed choices.

In essence, early intervention is not about rushing into a sea of unknowns. It's about embracing the knowns and leveraging them to your advantage. By dispelling myths about delaying diagnosis, we acknowledge the transformative power of early intervention in navigating the landscape of Parkinson's.

CHAPTER 3

Building Your Wellness Arsenal: Traditional Therapies

Exploring Deep Brain Stimulation (DBS) and Other Surgical Interventions: Potential Benefits and Considerations

Let's take a closer look at Deep Brain Stimulation (DBS) and other surgical interventions in the realm of Parkinson's treatment. While medications often take center stage, surgical options like DBS offer an alternative path that can significantly impact quality of life. Join me as we explore the potential benefits and considerations associated with these surgical interventions.

Deep Brain Stimulation (DBS): A Surgical Symphony

DBS is like fine-tuning an instrument in an orchestra – it's about precision and harmony. During DBS surgery, electrodes are implanted into specific areas of the brain responsible for movement control. These electrodes deliver electrical impulses, effectively modulating abnormal brain signals associated with Parkinson's symptoms.

Potential Benefits of DBS:

- Symptom Control: DBS can provide significant relief from motor symptoms, including tremors, rigidity, and dyskinesias, allowing for improved mobility and function.
- Medication Reduction: With successful DBS, some individuals may be able to reduce their reliance on Parkinson's medications, minimizing side effects associated with long-term use.
- Enhanced Quality of Life: By reducing motor fluctuations and dyskinesias, DBS can enhance overall quality of life, enabling individuals to engage in daily activities more freely.
- Long-Term Management: DBS offers a durable treatment option, with benefits often sustained over the long term, providing stability in symptom control.

- Flexibility and Adjustability: The settings of the DBS device can be adjusted non-invasively, allowing for personalized optimization of symptom control as the condition progresses.

Considerations and Challenges: Navigating the Surgical Landscape

While DBS holds promise, it's essential to approach it with careful consideration and awareness of potential challenges.

- Surgical Risks: Like any surgical procedure, DBS carries inherent risks, including infection, bleeding, and adverse reactions to anesthesia. However, with proper pre-operative evaluation and skilled surgical teams, these risks can be minimized.
- Post-Surgical Adjustments: Following DBS surgery, there is a period of adjustment as the settings of the device are optimized for optimal symptom control. Patience and collaboration with healthcare providers are key during this phase.
- Non-Motor Symptoms: While DBS primarily targets motor symptoms, it may not address non-motor aspects of Parkinson's, such as cognitive changes or mood

disorders. These aspects may require additional management strategies.

- Device-related Complications: Over time, complications such as electrode migration or battery depletion may arise, requiring further surgical intervention or device replacement.
- Patient Selection and Expectations: Not all individuals with Parkinson's are suitable candidates for DBS, and expectations should be realistic regarding the extent of symptom improvement achievable with surgery.

Exploring Other Surgical Interventions

In addition to DBS, other surgical interventions may be considered in certain cases, such as:

- Lesioning Procedures: These involve creating targeted lesions in specific brain regions to alleviate symptoms. While less commonly performed than DBS, they may be appropriate in select cases.
- Focused Ultrasound: This non-invasive procedure uses ultrasound waves to create lesions in targeted brain areas, offering a potential alternative to traditional surgical approaches.

- Gene Therapy: Emerging research explores the potential of gene therapy to modify the underlying disease process in Parkinson's, offering a novel approach to treatment.

Surgical interventions like DBS offer a valuable addition to the Parkinson's treatment arsenal, providing significant symptom relief and enhancing quality of life for many individuals. However, careful consideration of the potential benefits and challenges is essential in navigating the surgical landscape.

Unleashing the Power of Movement: Physical Therapy and Exercise for Parkinson's

Let's embark on a journey exploring the transformative impact of physical therapy and exercise in navigating the landscape of Parkinson's. In this dynamic duo, we discover not just routines and repetitions but a profound journey beyond limitations, where the power of movement becomes a beacon of strength and resilience.

Physical Therapy: A Personalized Compass

Physical therapy is akin to having a trusted guide on your journey. A skilled physical therapist assesses your unique challenges, tailoring exercises to address specific motor symptoms. It's not just about movement; it's about targeted and purposeful actions that unlock the potential for improved mobility and functionality.

Benefits of Physical Therapy:

- Enhanced Mobility: Targeted exercises can mitigate stiffness and rigidity, enhancing overall mobility and making daily tasks more manageable.
- Balance and Coordination: Parkinson's can impact balance, but physical therapy hones in on exercises that improve coordination and stability, reducing the risk of falls.
- Posture Improvement: Maintaining good posture is a subtle yet impactful aspect of physical well-being. Physical therapy addresses postural issues, promoting better alignment and reducing discomfort.
- Pain Management: Certain exercises and stretches can alleviate muscular discomfort and pain, contributing to an improved quality of life.
- Speech and Swallowing Improvement: For those facing speech and swallowing challenges, physical therapy can include exercises that strengthen relevant muscles, fostering improved communication and nutrition.

Exercise: The Elixir of Well-being

Exercise, in the context of Parkinson's, is not a mere routine but a powerful elixir that permeates various facets of health. Engaging in regular physical activity is a proactive step towards embracing the potential for a fulfilling life beyond the constraints of the condition.

Types of Exercise for Parkinson's:

- Aerobic Exercise: Activities like walking, cycling, or swimming promote cardiovascular health, improve endurance, and elevate mood.
- Strength Training: Building and maintaining muscle strength is crucial. Simple resistance exercises using weights or resistance bands contribute to overall well-being.
- Flexibility Exercises: Stretching routines enhance flexibility, reduce muscle stiffness, and support a fuller range of motion.
- Balance Exercises: Targeted exercises that challenge balance, such as tai chi or yoga, contribute to stability and reduce the risk of falls.

- Dance Therapy: Incorporating elements of dance not only provides physical benefits but also adds an element of joy and creativity to the exercise routine.

The Mind-Body Connection: Mindful Movement

Beyond the physical realm, there's a profound mind-body connection embedded in the power of movement. Mindful practices, such as tai chi or yoga, not only enhance physical well-being but also contribute to stress reduction and mental resilience.

Incorporating Mindfulness:

- Breath Awareness: Mindful attention to breath during exercises enhances relaxation and promotes a sense of calm.
- Focused Movements: Mindful engagement with each movement fosters a deeper connection between the body and mind.
- Stress Reduction: Regular exercise, coupled with mindfulness, becomes a potent tool in mitigating stress, a common companion in the Parkinson's journey.

Collaboration with Healthcare Providers: A Team Approach

Engaging in physical therapy and exercise is not a solitary endeavor but a collaborative effort with your healthcare team. Communication is key. Share your experiences, challenges, and goals with your physical therapist and healthcare provider. They become integral partners in tailoring a plan that aligns with your unique needs and aspirations.

Embracing the Journey: Beyond Limitations

As we embrace the journey of physical therapy and exercise in the realm of Parkinson's, let's redefine the narrative. It's not just about movements; it's about reclaiming a sense of agency, discovering the resilience within, and moving beyond perceived limitations. The power of movement becomes a transformative force, shaping a path towards a life filled with vitality and well-being.

Optimizing Life Through Occupational Therapy: Tailoring Daily Activities for Your Well-being

Occupational Therapy emerges as a personalized guide, offering a roadmap to adapt daily activities for optimal living. Let's explore this journey together, discovering not just routines but a customized approach to reclaiming a sense of purpose and independence in your daily life.

Understanding Occupational Therapy: Crafting Your Blueprint

Occupational therapy is not about changing who you are but about adapting your environment and routines to align with your unique needs. It's like crafting a personalized blueprint that enhances your ability to engage in meaningful activities, fostering independence and well-being.

Key Elements of Occupational Therapy:

Activity Analysis: An occupational therapist keenly observes your daily activities, breaking them down into manageable components. It's about understanding the intricacies of tasks, from getting dressed to preparing a meal.

- Environment Modification: Your living space becomes a canvas for adaptation. Simple modifications, like rearranging furniture or adding handrails, can make a significant impact on daily tasks.
- Assistive Devices: Occupational therapists guide you in selecting and using assistive devices tailored to your needs. These devices become tools of empowerment, aiding in tasks that may pose challenges.

- Energy Conservation Techniques: Parkinson's can affect energy levels. Occupational therapy introduces strategies to conserve energy, allowing you to accomplish more without unnecessary fatigue.
- Adaptive Strategies: From innovative techniques for buttoning a shirt to alternative approaches for cooking, occupational therapy introduces adaptive strategies that suit your unique abilities.

Step-by-Step Approach: Navigating Daily Activities

Let's embark on a step-by-step exploration of how occupational therapy can enhance specific daily activities, promoting a user-friendly and engaging experience for individuals with Parkinson's.

Activity: Getting Dressed

- Seated Dressing: Begin by sitting on the edge of your bed or a sturdy chair. This minimizes the challenge of maintaining balance while dressing.
- Use of Adaptive Clothing: Consider clothing with features like Velcro closures or magnetic buttons, easing the process of dressing independently.

- Breaking Down Steps: Divide the dressing routine into smaller, manageable steps. For example, focus on putting on one item of clothing at a time.
- Assistive Devices: Utilize dressing aids, such as long-handled reachers or sock aids, to extend your reach and make the process more accessible.

Activity: Meal Preparation

- Kitchen Organization: Arrange frequently used items at accessible heights. This reduces the need to reach or bend, making the kitchen a more user-friendly space.
- Adaptive Utensils: Explore utensils with ergonomic handles or built-up grips for easier handling during food preparation.
- Stool or Chair Use: Integrate short breaks during meal preparation by using a sturdy stool or chair. This helps manage fatigue and promotes comfort.
- Safety Measures: Consider non-slip mats, easy-grip kitchen tools, and strategically placed handrails to enhance safety while cooking.

Customizing Your Approach: A Holistic Perspective

Occupational therapy isn't just a set of instructions; it's a holistic approach to enhancing your overall well-being. It's about finding joy and fulfillment in the activities that matter most to you.

Tailoring Your Approach:

- Identifying Priorities: Work with your occupational therapist to identify the activities that hold the utmost significance in your daily life.
- Setting Realistic Goals: Establish achievable goals that align with your abilities and aspirations. Celebrate small victories along the way.
- Family and Caregiver Involvement: Collaborate with loved ones to integrate adaptations seamlessly into your daily routines. Their support can be invaluable.
- Regular Assessment and Adjustments: Parkinson's is dynamic, and your needs may evolve. Regular assessments with your occupational therapist ensure that adaptations remain effective and aligned with your current abilities.

As we navigate the landscape of occupational therapy together, let's embrace the potential for positive change in daily activities. It's not just about adapting; it's about reclaiming a sense of autonomy, fostering independence, and ensuring that every day is an opportunity for meaningful engagement.

CHAPTER 4

Beyond Medications: Exploring Complementary and Alternative Therapies

---

Harmony Within: Nurturing Well-being through Mind-Body Approaches

Embarking on a journey into the understanding of mind-body approaches opens the door to a sanctuary where stress management and well-being become not just aspirations but tangible realities. Join me as we explore the profound simplicity of mindfulness, meditation, and yoga – powerful tools accessible to all, weaving tranquility into the fabric of daily life.

The Essence of Mind-Body Connection: A Holistic Path

Picture the mind and body as intertwined companions, each influencing the other in a dance of harmony. Mind-body approaches recognize this connection, offering pathways to cultivate a serene state of being amidst the bustling demands of life.

MINDFULNESS: Embracing the Present Moment

Mindfulness is akin to a gentle anchor, grounding you in the present moment. It's about fostering awareness without judgment, allowing thoughts and sensations to come and go like ripples in a serene pond.

Incorporating Mindfulness into Daily Life:

- Breath Awareness: Start with simple breath awareness exercises. Inhale deeply, feel the air fill your lungs, and exhale slowly. This mindful breathing can be practiced anywhere, anytime.
- Daily Rituals: Infuse mindfulness into routine activities. Whether sipping your morning coffee or walking to the mailbox, engage your senses fully in the experience.
- Mindful Eating: During meals, savor each bite. Notice the flavors, textures, and sensations. This not only

enhances your eating experience but also promotes mindful awareness.

- Body Scan Meditation: Lie down comfortably, and mentally scan each part of your body, releasing tension as you go. This simple practice promotes relaxation and body-mind connection.

MEDITATION: Cultivating Inner Calm

Meditation is your sanctuary of stillness, a practice that cultivates a quiet space within. It's not about emptying the mind but about observing thoughts with a gentle curiosity and finding repose in the midst of life's whirlwind.

Starting Your Meditation Journey:

- Find a Quiet Space: Choose a quiet corner where you won't be disturbed. Sit comfortably, either on a chair or on the floor with a cushion to support your posture.
- Focus on the Breath: Direct your attention to the natural rhythm of your breath. Inhale and exhale gently, allowing your breath to guide you into a state of tranquility.
- Guided Meditations: Explore guided meditations available online or through apps. These provide gentle

prompts, making meditation more accessible, especially for beginners.

- Mindful Walking: Meditation doesn't always mean sitting still. Take a mindful walk, paying attention to each step and the sensations of movement.

YOGA: Uniting Body and Mind in Motion

Yoga is a symphony of movement and stillness, a practice that unites breath with intentional postures. It's not about contorting the body but about embracing a journey of self-discovery through gentle, deliberate movements.

Integrating Yoga into Your Routine:

- Start with Basics: Begin with simple yoga poses. Gentle stretches like the cat-cow pose or child's pose provide a foundation for building flexibility and body awareness.
- Focus on Breath: In yoga, breath is the guide. Coordinate your breath with each movement. Inhale as you reach, exhale as you fold. This synchronization enhances mindfulness.
- Online Classes or Apps: If you're new to yoga, consider online classes or apps offering beginner-friendly

sessions. Follow along at your own pace, embracing the joy of movement.

- Modify Poses as Needed: Yoga is about meeting your body where it is. Don't hesitate to modify poses to suit your comfort and abilities. The journey is yours, and every pose is a step towards well-being.

Weaving Mind-Body Practices into Your Tapestry

As you weave mindfulness, meditation, and yoga into the fabric of your daily life, remember that the essence lies in simplicity. These practices are not reserved for experts or those seeking enlightenment; they are tools for everyone, adaptable to your unique journey.

Keys to Incorporating Mind-Body Practices:

- Consistency over Intensity: Regular, brief practices trump sporadic, lengthy sessions. Consistency is the key to reaping the benefits of mind-body approaches.
- Personalization: Tailor these practices to suit your preferences and comfort. Your mindfulness, meditation, and yoga are uniquely yours.
- Gentle Self-Compassion: Approach these practices with gentleness. There's no judgment in this journey; it's

about embracing each moment with kindness towards yourself.

- Integration into Daily Life: Let these practices become companions in your daily routine. Whether it's a mindful breath during a meeting or a brief yoga stretch before bed, integration fosters sustainable well-being.

In the simplicity of mindfulness, meditation, and yoga, you hold the key to a harmonious existence. As you embark on this journey, relish the gentle moments, savor the tranquility, and discover the profound well-being that arises from within.

Nourishing the Mind: A Journey into Nutritional Considerations for Brain Health

Embarking on a path to support your brain health through nutrition is like tending to a garden – it requires care, attention, and a thoughtful approach. Join me as we explore the realm of dietary strategies, demystifying the process to make it not only accessible but an engaging journey towards enhanced well-being.

Understanding the Link: Nutrition and Brain Health
The connection between what we eat and how our brain functions is profound. Think of your brain as a powerhouse,

and the nutrients you consume as the fuel that keeps it running smoothly. Let's delve into the fundamental aspects of nutritional considerations for optimal brain health.

Key Nutrients for Brain Health:

- Omega-3 Fatty Acids: These are like the building blocks for your brain cells. Found in fatty fish, flaxseeds, and walnuts, omega-3s play a crucial role in cognitive function and mood regulation.
- Antioxidants: Think of antioxidants as the superheroes protecting your brain from oxidative stress. Brightly colored fruits and vegetables, such as berries, spinach, and kale, are rich sources of these defenders.
- Vitamins and Minerals: B-vitamins, vitamin D, and minerals like iron and zinc are essential for various brain functions. Whole grains, lean meats, dairy, and leafy greens are reliable sources.
- Hydration: Not a nutrient per se, but staying hydrated is vital. Picture water as the lubricant that keeps the gears of your cognitive machinery running smoothly.

Practical Steps for Brain-Boosting Nutrition: A User-Friendly Guide

Now, let's break down the process into actionable steps, making brain-boosting nutrition a tangible and achievable endeavor.

Step 1: Include Fatty Fish in Your Diet

Why? Fatty fish, such as salmon, trout, and sardines, are rich in omega-3 fatty acids, particularly DHA (docosahexaenoic acid), a crucial component of brain cell membranes.

How? Aim to include fatty fish in your meals at least twice a week. Grilled salmon, a tuna salad, or sardines on whole-grain crackers are delightful and brain-nourishing choices.

Step 2: Color Your Plate with Antioxidant-Rich Foods

Why? Antioxidants combat oxidative stress, reducing inflammation and supporting overall brain health.

How? Integrate a variety of colorful fruits and vegetables into your meals. Berries, dark leafy greens, and colorful bell peppers are not only visually appealing but also nutritionally dense.

Step 3: Prioritize Whole Grains and Lean Proteins

Why? Whole grains provide a steady supply of energy, while lean proteins contribute to the synthesis of neurotransmitters, essential for communication between brain cells.

How? Opt for whole grains like quinoa, brown rice, and oats. Include lean proteins such as poultry, fish, tofu, or legumes in your meals for a balanced nutritional profile.

Step 4: Stay Hydrated Throughout the Day

Why? Dehydration can impair cognitive function and concentration, emphasizing the importance of maintaining adequate fluid levels.

How? Make it a habit to sip water throughout the day. Consider infusing water with slices of citrus fruits or cucumber for added flavor and hydration appeal.

Step 5: Moderation and Variety

Why? A diverse and balanced diet ensures you receive a spectrum of nutrients, promoting overall brain health.

How? Embrace moderation and variety in your food choices. Explore different cuisines, try new recipes, and savor the rich tapestry of flavors and nutrients available.

Cooking Tips for Brain-Boosting Meals: A Culinary Adventure

Transforming these nutritional considerations into delicious meals involves creativity and a touch of culinary exploration. Let's embark on a culinary adventure with practical cooking tips:

- Omega-3 Packed Salad: Create a vibrant salad with leafy greens, berries, and a sprinkle of walnuts or flaxseeds. Drizzle with olive oil for an extra dose of brain-loving omega-3s.
- Quinoa Power Bowl: Build a nourishing bowl with cooked quinoa, colorful vegetables, and grilled salmon or chickpeas. Top it off with a lemon-tahini dressing for a delightful brain-boosting meal.
- Smoothie Delight: Blend together a refreshing smoothie using a base of Greek yogurt, a handful of berries, and a spoonful of chia seeds. This nutrient-packed smoothie is a quick and tasty brain pick-me-up.
- Baked Fish Fiesta: Explore different herbs and spices to create flavorful baked fish dishes. Herbs like rosemary

and thyme not only add zest but also contribute antioxidant properties.

The journey towards optimal brain health through nutrition is a blend of simplicity and creativity. By embracing these practical steps and culinary adventures, you are not just nourishing your brain but also cultivating a foundation for a flourishing and vibrant life.

Unlocking Vitality: A Guide to Optimal Sleep for Individuals with Parkinson's

Embarking on the quest for quality sleep is not just a necessity; it's a foundational pillar for vitality and cognitive well-being, especially for those navigating Parkinson's. In this exploration, we'll unravel the essentials of sleep hygiene – a practical approach tailored to enhance energy levels and cognitive function. Join me as we delve into straightforward strategies for a restful night's sleep.

Understanding the Sleep-Health Connection

Quality sleep is a linchpin for overall health, impacting energy, mood, and cognitive sharpness. For individuals with Parkinson's, optimizing sleep becomes even more crucial, considering the interplay between sleep quality and the challenges posed by the condition.

Key Aspects of Sleep Hygiene for Parkinson's:

- Consistent Sleep Schedule: Your body thrives on routine. Establishing a consistent sleep schedule, going to bed and waking up at the same time each day, helps regulate your internal clock.

- Create a Comfortable Sleep Environment: Transform your bedroom into a sanctuary of serenity. Ensure a comfortable mattress and pillows, adjust room temperature, and minimize noise and light to create an ideal sleep haven.

- Mindful Evening Routine: Engage in calming activities before bedtime. This could include reading a book, gentle stretching, or practicing relaxation techniques to signal to your body that it's time to wind down.

- Limit Stimulants and Screen Time: Caffeine and electronic devices can disrupt sleep. Aim to reduce caffeine intake in the evening, and avoid screens at least an hour before bedtime, as the blue light emitted can interfere with melatonin production.

Practical Steps for a Restful Night's Sleep: A User-Friendly Approach

Now, let's break down these key aspects into actionable steps, guiding you through a user-friendly approach to improve your sleep hygiene.

Step 1: Set Your Sleep Schedule

Why? Consistency reinforces your body's internal clock, promoting better sleep quality.

How? Choose a bedtime that allows for 7-9 hours of sleep and stick to it, even on weekends. Consistency reinforces your body's natural sleep-wake cycle.

Step 2: Optimize Your Sleep Environment

Why? A comfortable and calming sleep environment sets the stage for quality rest.

How? Invest in a comfortable mattress and pillows. Adjust room temperature to your preference and minimize noise and light. Consider blackout curtains for enhanced darkness.

Step 3: Wind Down Mindfully

Why? A mindful evening routine signals to your body that it's time to transition into a restful state.

How? Engage in activities that promote relaxation, such as reading a book, practicing gentle stretches, or listening to calming music. Avoid stimulating activities or heavy meals close to bedtime.

Step 4: Manage Stimulants and Screen Time

Why? Caffeine and screens can interfere with your ability to fall asleep and stay asleep.

How? Limit caffeine intake in the afternoon and evening. Create a screen-free zone at least an hour before bedtime to allow your brain to naturally wind down.

Step 5: Embrace a Consistent Wake-Up Time

Why? Consistency in waking up reinforces your body's natural circadian rhythm.

How? Set a consistent wake-up time, even on weekends. Exposure to natural light in the morning can further regulate your sleep-wake cycle.

Additional Tips for Improved Sleep:

- Regular Exercise: Incorporate regular physical activity into your routine, but aim to finish exercising a few hours before bedtime.
- Limit Naps: If you find the need to nap during the day, keep it short (20-30 minutes) and earlier in the day.
- Mind-Body Techniques: Explore relaxation techniques, such as deep breathing or progressive muscle relaxation, to calm your mind and body.
- Evaluate Medications: Consult with your healthcare provider to review medications that might impact sleep and discuss potential adjustments.

In the simplicity of consistent routines and mindful practices, you hold the key to unlocking the rejuvenating power of sleep. By incorporating these user-friendly steps into your daily life, you pave the way for improved energy levels, enhanced cognitive function, and a sense of vitality that resonates throughout your waking hours.

Holistic Well-being: Exploring Complementary Therapies for Parkinson's

Complementary therapies, such as massage, acupuncture, and other gentle modalities, weave a tapestry of holistic support for individuals navigating Parkinson's. Join me as we navigate through these therapeutic avenues, addressing concerns, and uncovering the potential benefits in a straightforward and engaging manner.

UNDERSTANDING COMPLEMENTARY THERAPIES: A Holistic Perspective

Complementary therapies are like gentle guides on your well-being journey, offering alternative approaches that complement traditional medical interventions. Let's explore two widely embraced therapies—massage and acupuncture—and touch upon other promising modalities.

MASSAGE: Unwinding Tensions and Nurturing the Body

Massage is more than a luxurious indulgence; it's a therapeutic tool that can address muscle stiffness, promote relaxation, and enhance overall well-being for individuals with Parkinson's.

Concerns:

- Muscle Rigidity: Individuals with Parkinson's often experience muscle stiffness. Massage, when done with care and tailored to individual needs, can alleviate tension without exacerbating rigidity.
- Sensory Sensitivity: Some may have heightened sensitivity. Communicating preferences and comfort levels with the massage therapist ensures a personalized and comfortable experience.

Potential Benefits:

- Improved Range of Motion: Gentle massage techniques can enhance flexibility and alleviate stiffness, promoting better range of motion.
- Stress Reduction: Massage is known to reduce stress and anxiety, contributing to an overall sense of relaxation.
- Enhanced Sleep Quality: The calming effects of massage can positively impact sleep patterns, fostering a more restful night.

ACUPUNCTURE: Balancing Energy for Wellness

Acupuncture, rooted in traditional Chinese medicine, involves the insertion of thin needles into specific points on the body to restore the flow of energy, or "qi."

Concerns:

Needle Sensitivity: Communicate any concerns about needle sensitivity with your acupuncturist. They can adjust techniques or explore alternatives such as acupressure.

Potential Benefits:

- Pain Management: Acupuncture may help manage pain, a common concern in Parkinson's, by stimulating the release of endorphins, the body's natural painkillers.
- Stress Reduction: Similar to massage, acupuncture can contribute to stress reduction and promote relaxation.
- Improved Sleep: Many individuals report improved sleep quality following acupuncture sessions.

Other Promising Complementary Approaches:

- Aromatherapy: Using essential oils to create a calming atmosphere. Lavender and chamomile are known for their relaxing properties.
- Music Therapy: Engaging with music to enhance mood and stimulate positive emotions.

- Tai Chi: A gentle form of exercise that combines movement and meditation, promoting balance and flexibility.

EXPLORING COMPLEMENTARY THERAPIES: A Step-by-Step Guide

Step 1: Assess Your Comfort Levels

Why? Understanding your comfort levels ensures a positive and personalized experience.

How? Communicate openly with the therapist or practitioner about any concerns or sensitivities you may have. They can tailor the session to accommodate your needs.

Step 2: Choose a Qualified Practitioner

Why? The expertise of the practitioner contributes to the safety and effectiveness of the therapy.

How? Research and choose practitioners who specialize in working with individuals with Parkinson's or those with experience in adaptive techniques.

Step 3: Set Realistic Expectations

Why? Having realistic expectations contributes to a positive and satisfying experience.

How? Understand that the effects of complementary therapies may vary. Some individuals may experience immediate benefits, while others may notice gradual improvements over time.

Step 4: Incorporate Complementary Therapies Into Your Routine

Why? Consistency is key to experiencing the potential benefits of complementary therapies.

How? Integrate sessions into your routine, whether it's a monthly massage or regular acupuncture appointments. Consistency enhances the cumulative effects.

In the realm of complementary therapies, the key lies in personalization and open communication. As you explore these gentle modalities, remember that each individual's experience is unique. Complementary therapies offer not only potential physical benefits but also moments of relaxation, rejuvenation, and a holistic approach to well-being.

CHAPTER 5

The Power of Your Network: Navigating Support Systems

Strength in Unity: Building Your Support Team for Parkinson's

Navigating Parkinson's is a journey that doesn't have to be solitary. In fact, it's strengthened by a robust support team, a collection of key players each contributing in their unique way. Join me as we explore the process of building a strong support team, identifying essential players and unraveling their roles in a clear, straightforward, and engaging manner.

UNDERSTANDING THE FOUNDATION: The Importance of a Support Team

Your support team is like a safety net, offering emotional, physical, and practical assistance. Recognizing the roles of each team member empowers you to build a foundation of strength, resilience, and shared understanding.

IDENTIFYING KEY PLAYERS AND THEIR ROLES: A Collaborative Guide

1. FAMILY AND FRIENDS: The Pillars of Emotional Support

- *Role*: Emotional anchors providing understanding, empathy, and companionship.
- *How:* Open communication is key. Share your experiences, fears, and triumphs. Encourage them to educate themselves about Parkinson's to foster a deeper understanding.

2. HEALTHCARE PROFESSIONALS: Your Expert Guides

- *Role:* The medical team offers professional guidance, treatment plans, and expert advice.
- *How:* Establish open communication. Actively participate in discussions about your treatment plan, ask questions, and seek clarification on any concerns.

3. PHYSICAL AND OCCUPATIONAL THERAPISTS: Enhancing Functionality

- ***Role:*** These professionals focus on improving physical and functional abilities, enhancing your quality of life.
- ***How:*** Engage actively in therapy sessions. Practice recommended exercises at home and communicate any challenges or progress.

4. SUPPORT GROUPS: A Community of Shared Experiences

- ***Role:*** Support groups offer a sense of belonging and understanding by connecting you with others facing similar challenges.
- ***How:*** Attend local or virtual support groups. Share your experiences, learn from others, and find encouragement in the collective strength of the community.

5. PATIENT ADVOCACY GROUPS: A Source of Resources and Connection

Role: Advocacy groups provide resources, information, and a platform for advocacy efforts.

How: Join reputable Parkinson's advocacy groups. Stay informed about research, treatment options, and available support resources.

BUILDING YOUR SUPPORT TEAM: A Step-by-Step Approach

Step 1: Self-Reflection

Why? Understanding your needs sets the foundation for building an effective support team.
How: Reflect on your daily challenges, emotional needs, and goals. Identify areas where support could make a significant difference.

Step 2: Identify Potential Team Members

Why? Recognizing potential team members ensures a comprehensive support structure.
How: Consider friends, family, healthcare professionals, therapists, support groups, and advocacy organizations. Assess how each could contribute to your support network.

Step 3: Open Communication

Why? Transparent communication fosters understanding and aligns everyone with a common goal.

How: Express your thoughts, feelings, and needs clearly. Encourage open dialogue with potential team members to establish a shared understanding.

Step 4: Set Expectations and Boundaries

Why? Clearly defined expectations ensure that everyone is on the same page.

How: Discuss roles, responsibilities, and boundaries with each team member. This includes clarifying how they can support you and any limitations they may have.

Step 5: Regular Check-Ins

Why? Regular check-ins maintain the strength and effectiveness of your support team.

How: Schedule regular updates with team members. Share updates on your health, discuss any adjustments needed, and express gratitude for their ongoing support.

Building a strong support team is not just a practical step; it's a transformative journey. Your team, united by understanding and shared goals, becomes a powerful force in navigating the challenges of Parkinson's. Remember, each member plays a unique role, contributing to a network of strength that empowers you to face each day with resilience.

Empowering Through Unity: Patient Advocacy Groups in the Parkinson's Community

Patient advocacy groups stand as beacons of connection and resources within the Parkinson's community, offering a sense of belonging and a wealth of knowledge. Join me as we explore the world of patient advocacy groups, unraveling their importance, and guiding you through the steps to find connection and resources.

UNDERSTANDING THE HEARTBEAT OF ADVOCACY GROUPS

Patient advocacy groups are like extended families, bringing together individuals on similar paths, creating a support network that transcends the challenges of Parkinson's. Let's delve into why these groups matter and how you can tap into their wealth of connection and resources.

FINDING CONNECTION: A Supportive Embrace

1. Shared Understanding:

Why: Patient advocacy groups provide a space where your experiences are understood.

How: Engage in discussions, share your journey, and listen to others. Recognize the common threads that weave your stories together.

2. Community Bonds:

Why: Being part of a community fosters a sense of belonging and shared strength.

How: Attend group events, whether in person or virtually. Participate in forums and connect with individuals who share similar experiences.

3. Emotional Support:

Why: The emotional support within advocacy groups can be a lifeline during challenging times.

How: Reach out to fellow members for support. Share your thoughts, fears, and triumphs, knowing that you are surrounded by a community that cares.

ACCESSING RESOURCES: A Wealth of Knowledge

1. Information Exchange:

Why: Advocacy groups are hubs of information, offering insights and updates on Parkinson's.

How: Actively participate in group discussions. Seek advice on treatment options, research updates, and practical tips for daily living.

2. Educational Opportunities:

Why: Advocacy groups often host educational events, empowering members with knowledge.

How: Attend workshops, webinars, or conferences organized by the group. Expand your understanding of Parkinson's and stay informed about the latest developments.

3. Advocacy Initiatives:

Why: These groups advocate for the Parkinson's community, influencing policy and promoting awareness.

How: Get involved in advocacy initiatives. Participate in awareness campaigns, share your story, and contribute to the collective effort to make a difference.

NAVIGATING PATIENT ADVOCACY GROUPS: A Step-by-Step Guide

Step 1: Identify Relevant Advocacy Groups

Why? Recognizing the right advocacy group aligns your needs with the offered support.

How: Research reputable Parkinson's advocacy groups. Consider factors such as the focus of the group, the accessibility of events, and the experiences shared by members.

Step 2: Join and Introduce Yourself

Why? Actively joining introduces you to the supportive environment and establishes your presence within the community.

How: Follow the group's joining process, whether online or through local chapters. Take a moment to introduce yourself, sharing a bit about your journey and what you hope to gain from the community.

Step 3: Engage in Discussions and Events

Why? Active engagement fosters connections and keeps you informed about valuable resources.

How: Participate in group discussions, forums, and events. Attend webinars or local meetings to connect with members and stay updated on relevant information.

Step 4: Seek and Offer Support

__Why?__ The reciprocal nature of support strengthens the community bonds.

__How:__ Don't hesitate to seek support when needed. Equally, offer support to others based on your experiences. The give-and-take builds a supportive ecosystem.

Step 5: Explore Advocacy Initiatives

__Why?__ Involvement in advocacy initiatives allows you to contribute to positive change for the Parkinson's community.

__How:__ Keep an eye on advocacy campaigns organized by the group. Contribute your voice, share your story, and actively participate in initiatives that align with your values.

Patient advocacy groups are not just entities; they are dynamic communities offering a collective journey of empowerment. As you step into this supportive realm, remember that your presence and experiences contribute to the shared strength of the Parkinson's community. In unity, there is strength, and in patient advocacy groups, there is a shared heartbeat that resonates with resilience and hope.

Navigating the Conversation: Effective Communication in the Parkinson's Journey

Communication lies at the heart of building understanding, whether with loved ones or healthcare providers. In the realm of Parkinson's, articulating your needs becomes a crucial skill. Join me as we explore communication tips, unveiling a roadmap that is clear, compassionate, and empowers both you and your support network.

Effective communication is a bridge that connects you with your loved ones and healthcare providers, fostering a shared understanding of your experiences, needs, and aspirations. Let's embark on this journey together, cultivating a communication style that transcends the challenges of Parkinson's.

COMMUNICATION TIPS FOR LOVED ONES: Nurturing Understanding

1. Initiate Open Dialogues:
Why: Openness lays the foundation for understanding.
How: Initiate conversations about your feelings, experiences, and any challenges you may be facing due to Parkinson's.

Encourage loved ones to share their thoughts and concerns as well.

2. Educate Without Overwhelming:

Why: Providing information helps dispel misconceptions.

How: Share educational resources about Parkinson's in a digestible manner. Focus on key aspects relevant to your journey, and be open to answering questions.

3. Express Your Emotional Needs:

Why: Emotional support is vital.

How: Communicate your emotional needs clearly. Whether you need a listening ear, a moment of understanding, or simply someone to share a laugh with, express those needs openly.

4. Use "I" Statements:

Why: "I" statements promote ownership of feelings.

How: Frame your thoughts using "I" statements to express your emotions and needs. For example, say, "I feel fatigued today, and I could use some support" instead of placing blame.

COMMUNICATION TIPS FOR HEALTHCARE PROVIDERS: Navigating Collaborative Care

1. Prepare for Appointments:

Why: Preparedness ensures you get the most from your appointments.

How: List your symptoms, questions, and concerns before appointments. This proactive approach helps you cover all relevant topics during your time with the healthcare provider.

2. Be Transparent About Symptoms:

Why: Clarity aids accurate diagnosis and treatment.

How: Clearly describe your symptoms, their frequency, and any patterns you've observed. Provide a comprehensive overview of your experiences to guide the healthcare provider in making informed decisions.

3. Ask Questions and Seek Clarifications:

Why: Understanding your treatment plan is crucial.

How: Don't hesitate to ask questions about medications, potential side effects, and the overall treatment plan. Seek clarifications to ensure you are actively involved in decisions about your care.

4. Share Updates on Lifestyle Changes:

Why: Lifestyle changes impact your well-being.

How: Inform your healthcare provider about any lifestyle modifications, such as dietary changes or new exercise routines. These details contribute to a holistic understanding of your health.

GUIDING THE CONVERSATION: A Step-by-Step Approach

Step 1: Self-Reflection

Why? Understanding your own needs sets the tone for effective communication.
How: Reflect on your emotional and physical needs. Identify key aspects you want to communicate to your loved ones and healthcare providers.

Step 2: Create a Communication Plan

Why? A plan ensures that you cover all essential topics during conversations.
How: List key points you want to communicate. This could include symptoms, emotional needs, or specific questions for healthcare providers.

Step 3: Initiate Open Dialogues

Why? Openness fosters understanding and empathy.

How: Start conversations with loved ones about your Parkinson's journey. Encourage them to share their thoughts and feelings as well.

Step 4: Practice "I" Statements

Why? "I" statements promote ownership and clarity.
How: Use "I" statements to express your emotions and needs. This helps avoid misunderstandings and encourages a supportive atmosphere.

Step 5: Prepare for Healthcare Appointments

Why? Preparedness ensures effective communication with healthcare providers.
How: List symptoms, questions, and concerns before appointments. This proactive approach ensures that you address all relevant topics during your appointments.

Step 6: Be Transparent and Seek Clarifications

Why? Clarity aids accurate diagnosis and treatment decisions.

How: Clearly describe symptoms to healthcare providers and ask questions about your treatment plan. Seek clarifications to actively engage in decisions about your care.

Step 7: Share Lifestyle Updates

Why? Lifestyle changes impact your well-being and should be communicated.

How: Inform healthcare providers about any lifestyle modifications you've made. These details contribute to a holistic understanding of your health.

In the realm of Parkinson's, effective communication is not just a skill; it's a powerful tool for empowerment. As you navigate conversations with loved ones and healthcare providers, remember that your voice matters. Each exchange is an opportunity to foster understanding, strengthen connections, and shape a collaborative journey towards well-being.

Navigating Emotional Waters: Managing Mental Health Concerns in the Parkinson's Journey

The emotional terrain of a Parkinson's journey can be challenging, and acknowledging and addressing mental health concerns is a crucial aspect of holistic well-being. Join me as we delve into the complexities of managing anxiety, depression, and other emotional challenges in a way that is clear, compassionate, and empowers both you and your support network.

Understanding the Emotional Landscape

Emotional well-being is an integral part of the Parkinson's journey. Managing anxiety, depression, and other mental health concerns requires a nuanced approach that considers the unique aspects of living with Parkinson's. Let's explore strategies that foster resilience and promote mental well-being.

MANAGING ANXIETY: A Step Towards Calmness

1. Identify Triggers:
Why: Understanding triggers helps in proactively managing anxiety.
How: Reflect on situations or factors that contribute to anxiety. This self-awareness is the first step towards developing coping strategies.

2. Breathing Exercises:

Why: Controlled breathing can alleviate anxiety symptoms.

How: Practice deep-breathing exercises. Inhale slowly, hold for a few seconds, and exhale gradually. This simple technique can help restore a sense of calmness.

3. Mindfulness Practices:

Why: Mindfulness promotes present-moment awareness, reducing anxiety.

How: Engage in mindfulness activities such as meditation or mindful walking. These practices anchor your focus in the present, easing anxious thoughts.

4. Create a Support System:

Why: Sharing feelings lessens the burden.

How: Open up to trusted loved ones about your anxiety. Knowing that you have a support system can provide comfort and understanding.

NAVIGATING DEPRESSION: Finding Light in Darkness

1. Establish a Routine:

Why: Routine fosters a sense of stability.

How: Create a daily schedule that includes activities you enjoy. This structure can provide a sense of purpose and contribute to mood improvement.

2. Physical Activity:

Why: Exercise releases endorphins, enhancing mood.

How: Engage in activities such as walking, gentle yoga, or tailored exercises. Find activities that bring joy and contribute to overall well-being.

3. Connect Socially:

Why: Social connections combat feelings of isolation.

How: Maintain social connections, whether through in-person or virtual interactions. Share your experiences with friends or join support groups to foster a sense of belonging.

4. Professional Support:

Why: Seeking professional help is a sign of strength.

How: Consult with a mental health professional, such as a psychologist or counselor. They can provide tailored strategies to navigate depression and offer support.

ADDRESSING SEX & INTIMACY: Nurturing Connection

1. Open Communication:

Why: Communication is key in maintaining intimacy.

How: Initiate open discussions with your partner about your feelings, concerns, and desires. Create a safe space for expressing emotions.

2. Adapt and Explore:

Why: Adaptation fosters continued intimacy.

How: Explore different ways to experience intimacy that accommodate physical changes. Focus on emotional connection and shared moments of closeness.

3. Involve Healthcare Professionals:

Why: Medical advice can offer guidance.

How: If physical challenges impact intimacy, consult with healthcare professionals. They can provide advice, recommend specialists, or suggest strategies to address specific concerns.

GUIDING THROUGH EMOTIONAL CHALLENGES: A Step-by-Step Approach

Step 1: Self-Reflection

Why? Understanding your emotional state is the foundation for effective management.

How: Reflect on your emotional well-being. Identify specific concerns such as anxiety, depression, or challenges related to intimacy.

Step 2: Identify Triggers and Concerns

Why? Identifying triggers provides insight into potential coping strategies.

How: List situations or factors that contribute to anxiety, depression, or concerns related to intimacy. This self-awareness helps in developing targeted approaches.

Step 3: Engage in Coping Strategies

Why? Implementing coping strategies empowers you to navigate emotional challenges.

How: Practice breathing exercises, engage in mindfulness practices, establish routines, and incorporate physical activities. Gradually introduce these strategies into your daily life.

Step 4: Communicate Openly

Why? Open communication strengthens relationships and fosters understanding.

How: Initiate honest conversations with loved ones about your emotional state. Share your thoughts, concerns, and feelings related to anxiety, depression, or intimacy. Create a supportive environment for dialogue.

Step 5: Seek Professional Support

Why? Professional guidance enhances the effectiveness of coping strategies.
How: Consult with mental health professionals for personalized strategies. If concerns about intimacy arise, involve healthcare professionals who specialize in addressing such matters.

Step 6: Explore and Adapt

Why? Adaptation is key to maintaining well-being in the face of challenges.
How: Explore new activities, adapt routines, and consider different approaches to maintain emotional and physical well-being. Embrace change as a dynamic part of your journey.

Step 7: Foster Social Connections

Why? Social connections combat feelings of isolation and contribute to overall well-being.

How: Actively participate in social interactions. Maintain connections with friends, family, and support groups. Share experiences and receive support from others who understand your journey.

Navigating emotional challenges in the Parkinson's journey requires a blend of self-awareness, coping strategies, and open communication. As you engage in this process, remember that seeking support is a strength, and each step you take towards emotional well-being is a testament to your resilience.

CHAPTER 6

Living Well, Not Just Managing: Redefining Your Quality of Life

---

Embracing Progress: Setting Realistic Goals and Celebrating Small Victories

In the journey of living with Parkinson's, setting realistic goals and celebrating small victories can be powerful tools for maintaining motivation, boosting confidence, and fostering a sense of accomplishment. Let's explore practical strategies for setting goals, tracking progress, and embracing every step forward with enthusiasm and resilience in a clear, relatable, and engaging manner.

Step 1: Defining Your Goals

Why? Setting clear goals provides direction and purpose in your Parkinson's journey.

How: Begin by reflecting on your aspirations and priorities. What do you hope to achieve in various aspects of your life, such as physical health, emotional well-being, relationships, hobbies, or personal development? Write down **S**pecific, **M**easurable, **A**chievable, **R**elevant, and **T**ime-bound (SMART) goals that align with your values and interests.

Step 2: Breaking Down Goals into Manageable Steps

Why? Breaking down goals into smaller steps makes them more attainable and manageable.

How: Once you've defined your overarching goals, identify the specific actions or milestones needed to reach them. Break down each goal into smaller, actionable steps that you can easily incorporate into your daily routine. For example, if your goal is to improve mobility, smaller steps could include scheduling regular physical therapy sessions, practicing daily exercises, or incorporating more movement into your daily activities.

Step 3: Tracking Progress and Adjusting Goals

Why? Monitoring progress allows you to stay on track and make necessary adjustments along the way.

How: Keep a journal or use a goal-tracking app to record your progress regularly. Celebrate the completion of each small step and acknowledge any setbacks or challenges with compassion and resilience. Periodically review your goals and adjust them as needed based on your evolving needs, priorities, and capabilities.

Step 4: Celebrating Small Victories

Why? Celebrating small victories boosts morale, enhances motivation, and reinforces positive behaviors.

How: Take time to acknowledge and celebrate every small accomplishment, no matter how minor it may seem. Whether it's completing a challenging exercise routine, achieving a personal milestone, or successfully managing a symptom, find ways to reward yourself and express gratitude for your progress. Share your achievements with loved ones or support groups to amplify the joy and encouragement.

Step 5: Cultivating a Growth Mindset

Why? Embracing a growth mindset fosters resilience and adaptability in the face of challenges.

How: Embrace the belief that challenges and setbacks are opportunities for growth and learning. View obstacles as temporary setbacks rather than insurmountable barriers. Practice self-compassion and positive self-talk, reframing setbacks as opportunities to learn, grow, and improve.

Step 6: Adjusting Goals as Needed

Why? Flexibility and adaptability are essential for navigating the ups and downs of living with Parkinson's.

How: Be open to adjusting your goals and expectations as your circumstances change. Recognize that progress may not always follow a linear path and that setbacks are a natural part of the journey. Stay flexible, resilient, and focused on continuous improvement rather than perfection.

Step 7: Seeking Support and Accountability

Why? Support from others can provide encouragement, motivation, and accountability.

How: Share your goals with trusted friends, family members, or support groups. Seek encouragement, advice, and accountability from individuals who understand and support your journey. Consider partnering with a coach, mentor, or accountability buddy to stay motivated and committed to your goals.

Setting realistic goals and celebrating small victories are essential practices for fostering resilience, maintaining motivation, and enhancing well-being in the face of Parkinson's. By defining clear goals, breaking them down into manageable steps, tracking progress, celebrating achievements, cultivating a growth mindset, and seeking support, you can embrace every step forward with enthusiasm and resilience.

Rediscovering Joy: Adapting Hobbies and Activities in the Parkinson's Journey

Engaging in hobbies and activities holds a special place in our lives, providing a source of joy, purpose, and fulfillment. In the context of Parkinson's, adapting these passions becomes an exploration of resilience and creativity. Let's embark on a journey together, discovering practical strategies for embracing your favorite pursuits in a way that aligns with the realities of living with Parkinson's.

Reimagining Hobbies: A Personal and Transformative Adventure

Adapting hobbies and activities in the face of Parkinson's disease is about rediscovering joy, maintaining connections to the things that bring fulfillment, and finding new ways to express your passions.

Step 1: Reflecting on Your Passions

Why? Reflection allows you to identify the core elements of your passions and hobbies.

How: Take a moment to reflect on the activities that have brought you joy and fulfillment throughout your life. What aspects of these pursuits resonate with you the most? Whether it's the creative expression, physical movement, or social connection, understanding the essence of your passions is the first step in adapting them to your current circumstances.

Step 2: Identifying Adaptations and Modifications

Why? Identifying adaptations ensures that your hobbies remain accessible and enjoyable.

How: Consider how you can modify your favorite activities to accommodate any physical or cognitive changes associated with Parkinson's. For example, if you enjoy painting but find fine motor skills challenging, explore larger brushes or adaptive tools. If gardening is your passion but mobility is a concern, consider raised beds or container gardening.

Step 3: Exploring New Avenues

Why? Exploring new avenues introduces variety and excitement into your adapted hobbies.

How: Be open to exploring new aspects of your passions. If you love music but playing instruments becomes challenging, consider exploring music appreciation, singing, or even experimenting with digital music software. The key is to maintain the spirit of your passions while embracing fresh and accessible approaches.

Step 4: Engaging in Social Hobbies

Why? Social engagement is a crucial component of well-being.

How: If your hobbies involve social interaction, such as book clubs, art classes, or game nights, find ways to adapt these activities for optimal enjoyment. Consider virtual options, flexible schedules, or smaller group settings to accommodate your needs and preferences.

Step 5: Embracing Mindful Enjoyment

Why? Mindful enjoyment ensures that your adapted hobbies become moments of presence and fulfillment.

How: Approach your adapted hobbies with mindfulness, focusing on the joy and satisfaction they bring rather than any limitations. Be fully present in the experience, savoring each moment and appreciating the positive impact these activities have on your overall well-being.

Step 6: Seeking Support and Connection

Why? Shared experiences and support enhance the enjoyment of adapted hobbies.

How: Connect with others who share similar adapted hobbies or explore support groups specifically focused on creative adaptations. Share your experiences, learn from others, and build a supportive community that understands the unique journey of adapting passions in the context of Parkinson's.

Step 7: Celebrating Milestones and Progress

Why? Celebrating milestones reinforces the positive impact of adapted hobbies on your well-being.

How: Acknowledge and celebrate the progress you make in adapting and enjoying your hobbies. Whether it's completing a project, learning a new skill, or simply finding renewed pleasure in a familiar activity, take time to reflect on your achievements and share these victories with your support network.

Adapting hobbies and activities in the face of Parkinson's is not a departure from joy; it's a dynamic and creative exploration of your passions. By reflecting on your core interests, identifying adaptations, exploring new avenues, engaging socially, embracing mindfulness, seeking support, and celebrating milestones, you weave a tapestry of joy that reflects the resilience and creativity within you.

Navigating the Journey: Travel Tips for the Parkinson's Explorer

Embarking on a journey, whether near or far, is a wonderful pursuit that should be accessible and enjoyable for everyone, including those living with Parkinson's. In this exploration of travel tips, let's delve into practical strategies and thoughtful considerations that can make your travel experiences not only possible but also enriching and memorable.

PREPARING FOR THE ADVENTURE: A Step-by-Step Guide to Traveling with Parkinson's

Traveling with Parkinson's requires a bit of extra planning and consideration, but with the right preparations, you can unlock the joy of exploration and create lasting memories.

Step 1: Assessing Your Comfort Level

Why? Understanding your comfort level sets the foundation for enjoyable travel.

How: Reflect on your current physical and cognitive abilities. Consider factors such as mobility, balance, stamina, and any specific symptoms you may experience. This self-assessment will help you tailor your travel plans to align with your individual needs and preferences.

Step 2: Choosing Suitable Destinations

Why? Selecting destinations that accommodate your needs enhances the overall travel experience.

How: Research and choose destinations that offer accessibility, medical facilities, and amenities that align with your requirements. Consider factors like climate, altitude, and terrain, and opt for places with a range of activities that match your interests and abilities.

Step 3: Planning Ahead for Accommodations

Why? Thoughtful accommodation planning ensures a comfortable and enjoyable stay.

How: Contact hotels or accommodations in advance to discuss your specific needs. Inquire about accessibility features, such as ramps, elevators, or ground-floor rooms. Communicate any specific requests related to Parkinson's symptoms, ensuring a more accommodating and stress-free stay.

Step 4: Packing Essentials for Comfort and Safety

Why? Packing essentials ensures you have everything you need for a smooth and secure journey.

How: Create a comprehensive packing list that includes medications, medical supplies, comfortable clothing, and any mobility aids you may require. Carry a copy of your medical information, including a list of medications and emergency contacts, to provide to healthcare professionals if needed.

Step 5: Planning Your Itinerary Mindfully

Why? A well-planned itinerary maximizes enjoyment while minimizing stress.

How: Plan your daily activities with breaks and downtime in mind. Allow flexibility in your schedule to accommodate any unexpected changes or variations in your energy levels. Consider shorter, more leisurely excursions to ensure a more relaxed pace.

Step 6: Staying Hydrated and Well-Nourished

Why? Proper hydration and nutrition contribute to overall well-being during travel.

How: Stay mindful of your water intake and carry a reusable water bottle to ensure hydration throughout the journey. Plan for regular, balanced meals, and include snacks that align with your dietary preferences and restrictions.

Step 7: Informing Travel Companions and Seeking Assistance

Why? Communication and support from travel companions enhance the overall travel experience.

How: Inform your travel companions about your specific needs and preferences. Discuss a plan for assistance if required, whether it's navigating crowded areas, helping with luggage, or providing emotional support. Open communication ensures everyone is on the same page and contributes to a more enjoyable journey.

Step 8: Embracing Mindful Moments During Travel

Why? Mindfulness enhances the travel experience by fostering presence and appreciation.

How: Take moments to savor the beauty of your surroundings, connect with the local culture, and engage in activities that bring you joy. Mindful practices, such as deep breathing or short meditation sessions, can also contribute to a sense of calm and well-being during your journey.

Step 9: Being Prepared for Medical Emergencies

Why? Preparedness for medical emergencies provides peace of mind.

How: Carry a small travel medical kit with essential medications, first-aid supplies, and any necessary medical documentation. Familiarize yourself with local healthcare facilities at your destination, and have a plan in place for seeking medical assistance if needed.

Step 10: Reflecting on the Journey and Celebrating Experiences

Why? Reflection and celebration contribute to the overall enjoyment and positive impact of your travel experiences.

How: Take time to reflect on the moments of joy, the people you've met, and the places you've explored. Celebrate the resilience and adaptability that allowed you to embark on this journey with Parkinson's, and acknowledge the personal growth and enrichment gained from the experience.

Traveling with Parkinson's is not just about reaching a destination; it's about embracing the journey with mindfulness, adaptability, and joy. By assessing your comfort level, choosing suitable destinations, planning accommodations, packing essentials, mindful itinerary planning, staying hydrated, informing travel companions, embracing mindfulness, preparing for emergencies, and reflecting on the journey, you can unveil the beauty of travel with Parkinson's and create cherished memories that last a lifetime.

Nurturing Connections: Overcoming Challenges in Intimacy and Relationships

Navigating intimacy and relationships while living with Parkinson's disease is a journey filled with unique challenges and opportunities for growth. In this exploration, I'll delve into practical strategies and heartfelt insights to help you foster connection, strengthen relationships, and embrace intimacy with confidence and resilience.

Embracing Connection: A Personal Exploration of Intimacy and Relationships

Intimacy and relationships are integral aspects of our lives, offering comfort, support, and joy. Yet, when Parkinson's enters the picture, maintaining these connections can present hurdles that require understanding, patience, and adaptability.

Understanding the Impact of Parkinson's on Relationships

Living with Parkinson's can affect various aspects of intimacy and relationships, from physical changes to emotional shifts. Symptoms such as tremors, rigidity, and fatigue may impact physical intimacy, while mood fluctuations and cognitive changes can influence emotional connections.

Step 1: Open Communication

Why? Communication forms the foundation of healthy relationships.

How: Foster open and honest communication with your partner about your feelings, needs, and concerns related to Parkinson's. Create a safe space for both of you to express yourselves without judgment or fear. Discuss how Parkinson's may be affecting your intimacy and explore ways to adapt together.

Step 2: Educating Your Partner

Why? Education promotes understanding and empathy.

How: Share information about Parkinson's with your partner, including symptoms, treatment options, and potential challenges. Encourage them to ask questions and seek resources to deepen their understanding of how Parkinson's may impact your relationship. Knowledge can help alleviate misconceptions and foster greater empathy and support.

Step 3: Embracing Physical Intimacy

Why? Physical intimacy is an important aspect of romantic relationships.

How: Explore ways to adapt physical intimacy to accommodate any challenges posed by Parkinson's symptoms. Experiment with different positions, pacing, and techniques that minimize discomfort and maximize pleasure for both partners. Remember that intimacy goes beyond sexual activity and can include affectionate touch, cuddling, and non-sexual physical closeness.

Step 4: Nurturing Emotional Connection

Why? Emotional connection strengthens the bond between partners.

How: Engage in activities that foster emotional intimacy, such as meaningful conversations, shared hobbies, and acts of kindness and appreciation. Practice active listening and empathy, validating each other's feelings and experiences. Find moments to connect on a deeper level and express your love and appreciation for one another.

Step 5: Seeking Support Together

Why? Support from each other and external resources can bolster your relationship.

How: Attend support groups or counseling sessions together to gain insights, coping strategies, and a sense of community from others facing similar challenges. Lean on each other for emotional support during difficult times and celebrate victories together, no matter how small. Remember that you're a team, facing Parkinson's together.

Step 6: Cultivating Connection Beyond Your Partner

Why? Connection with others enriches your life and strengthens your support network.

How: Maintain connections with friends, family members, and community groups to ensure a diverse support network. Participate in social activities together, such as group outings, game nights, or volunteer work. Strengthening connections outside of your romantic relationship can provide additional sources of support and fulfillment.

Step 7: Embracing Adaptability and Resilience

Why? Adaptability and resilience are essential qualities for navigating challenges together.

How: Approach Parkinson's as a shared journey, recognizing that both partners may need to adapt and evolve over time. Embrace flexibility and creativity in finding solutions to challenges, and celebrate your resilience in overcoming obstacles together. Remember that facing challenges as a team can strengthen your bond and deepen your connection.

Maintaining intimacy and relationships while living with Parkinson's requires patience, understanding, and a willingness to adapt. By fostering open communication, educating your partner, embracing physical and emotional intimacy, seeking support together, cultivating connections beyond your partnership, and embracing adaptability and resilience, you can navigate the challenges of Parkinson's while fostering a deep and meaningful connection with your partner.

CHAPTER 7

Advocating for Yourself: Taking Charge of Your Healthcare

Empowering Your Journey: Asking Informed Questions in Parkinson's Treatment Decisions

Making informed decisions about your Parkinson's treatment is a proactive and empowering step on your journey. In this exploration, I'll delve into the art of asking informed questions, guiding you through a step-by-step process that will help you engage actively in your treatment decisions with confidence and clarity.

TAKING THE REINS: A Step-by-Step Guide to Informed Treatment Decisions

Empowering yourself in the decision-making process involves understanding your treatment options, communicating effectively with your healthcare team, and actively participating in decisions that impact your well-being.

Step 1: Educate Yourself about Parkinson's and Treatment Options

Why? Knowledge is the foundation of informed decision-making.

How: Invest time in learning about Parkinson's disease, its progression, and the available treatment options. Explore reputable sources, attend educational sessions, and engage with patient advocacy groups to deepen your understanding. This foundational knowledge will serve as a crucial tool when discussing treatment choices with your healthcare team.

Step 2: Create a List of Questions

Why? A prepared list ensures you cover all your concerns during appointments.

How: Before your appointments, compile a list of questions related to your condition, potential treatments, and any other aspects that you would like to address. Consider both general questions about Parkinson's and specific inquiries about treatment options, side effects, and lifestyle adjustments.

Step 3: Prioritize Your Questions

Why? Prioritization ensures that the most crucial questions are addressed.

How: Arrange your list of questions in order of importance. Start with inquiries about critical aspects of your treatment and well-being. This ensures that even if time is limited during appointments, you address the most crucial concerns first.

Step 4: Seek Clarification on Medical Jargon

Why? Clear communication enhances understanding and decision-making.

How: If you encounter medical jargon or terms you don't fully understand, don't hesitate to ask your healthcare team for clarification. Understanding the language used in discussions about your treatment is essential for making informed decisions.

Step 5: Discuss Treatment Goals and Expectations

Why? Aligning treatment goals ensures a shared understanding with your healthcare team.

How: Engage in a conversation with your healthcare provider about the goals of your Parkinson's treatment. Discuss what you hope to achieve, whether it's symptom management, improved quality of life, or specific functional goals. Ensure that your expectations align with the realistic outcomes of the chosen treatment plan.

Step 6: Explore Alternatives and Potential Risks

Why? Considering alternatives and risks provides a comprehensive view of your options.

How: Discuss alternative treatment approaches with your healthcare team, and inquire about potential risks and benefits. Having a thorough understanding of the potential outcomes, as well as any associated risks, allows you to make decisions that align with your preferences and values.

Step 7: Engage in Shared Decision-Making

Why? Shared decision-making ensures collaboration between you and your healthcare team.

How: Actively participate in the decision-making process by expressing your preferences, concerns, and priorities. Discuss the information you've gathered, ask for your healthcare provider's insights, and work together to formulate a treatment plan that suits your individual needs.

Step 8: Request Written Information

Why? Written information serves as a valuable resource for ongoing reference.

How: Ask your healthcare team for written materials or resources that detail your treatment plan, including medications, potential side effects, and lifestyle recommendations. Having this information in writing allows you to review and reference it at your own pace.

Step 9: Schedule Follow-Up Appointments

Why? Follow-up appointments ensure ongoing communication and adjustments to your treatment plan.

How: Schedule regular follow-up appointments with your healthcare team to assess the effectiveness of your treatment, address any concerns or changes in symptoms, and make adjustments as needed. Regular check-ins maintain an open line of communication and allow for ongoing collaboration in your care.

HERE IS A LIST OF IMPORTANT QUESTIONS PEOPLE WITH PARKINSON'S DISEASE CAN ASK THEIR HEALTHCARE PROVIDER:

Understanding Parkinson's Disease:

1. What stage of Parkinson's disease am I currently in?
2. Can you explain how Parkinson's disease progresses over time?
3. What specific symptoms of Parkinson's should I be aware of and monitor?

Treatment Options:

4. What medications are commonly prescribed for Parkinson's, and how do they work?
5. Are there any new medications or therapies that might be suitable for my condition?
6. How will the prescribed medications help manage my symptoms, and what are the potential side effects?

Lifestyle and Diet:

7. Are there specific lifestyle changes I should consider to better manage my symptoms?

8. How can diet and nutrition play a role in managing Parkinson's disease?

Physical and Occupational Therapy:

9. How can physical therapy benefit me in managing the physical symptoms of Parkinson's?

10. Are there specific exercises or physical activities that you recommend for my condition?

11. Can occupational therapy help me adapt daily activities to my changing abilities?

Deep Brain Stimulation (DBS) and Surgical Options:

12. What is Deep Brain Stimulation (DBS), and how might it benefit someone with Parkinson's?

13. What are the potential risks and benefits of surgical interventions for Parkinson's?

Mental Health and Emotional Well-being:

14. How can Parkinson's disease impact my mental health and emotional well-being?

15. Are there support groups or counseling services available to help cope with the emotional aspects of Parkinson's?

Clinical Trials and Research:

16. Are there any ongoing clinical trials or research studies that I might be eligible for?
17. How can participating in clinical trials contribute to advancing Parkinson's research?

Cognitive Impacts:

18. Are there cognitive aspects of Parkinson's disease that I should be aware of?
19. What strategies can help manage cognitive changes associated with Parkinson's?

Sleep Disturbances:

20. How does Parkinson's disease affect sleep, and what can be done to improve sleep quality?

Medication Management:

21. How often should I take my medications, and what is the best way to manage any potential side effects?

22. Are there any interactions between Parkinson's medications and other medications I may be taking?

Mobility and Falls:

23. How can I address mobility issues and reduce the risk of falls associated with Parkinson's?

24. Are there assistive devices or mobility aids that might benefit me?

Driving and Transportation:

25. Are there any restrictions or considerations regarding my ability to drive with Parkinson's?

26. What alternative transportation options are available for individuals with Parkinson's?

Genetic Factors:

27. Is Parkinson's disease influenced by genetic factors, and should I consider genetic testing?

Work and Employment:

28. How might Parkinson's disease impact my ability to work, and are there accommodations available?

29. Are there resources or support services for individuals with Parkinson's who are still working?

Pain Management:

30. Can Parkinson's disease cause pain, and how can it be managed?

Vision and Hearing:

31. Are there vision or hearing issues associated with Parkinson's, and how can they be addressed?

Dental Health:

32. Are there specific dental considerations for individuals with Parkinson's disease?

Balance and Coordination:

33. What exercises or activities can help improve balance and coordination?

Travel Considerations:

34. Are there any specific considerations or precautions I should take when traveling with Parkinson's?

Alternative Therapies:

35. Can complementary and alternative therapies, such as acupuncture or massage, benefit Parkinson's symptoms?

Communication with Healthcare Providers:

36. How frequently should I schedule follow-up appointments, and what should be discussed during these visits?
37. Are there warning signs or symptoms that warrant immediate medical attention?

Advance Directives and Long-Term Planning:

38. When is it appropriate to discuss advance directives and long-term care planning?
39. What resources are available for long-term care and support?

40. How can family members and caregivers best support someone with Parkinson's disease, and are there resources available for them?

These questions provide a starting point for individuals with Parkinson's to engage in meaningful discussions with their healthcare providers, empowering them to actively participate in their care and make informed decisions about their well-being.

Asking informed questions is not just a part of the treatment process; it's a powerful tool that puts you at the center of your Parkinson's journey.

By educating yourself, creating a list of questions, prioritizing concerns, seeking clarification, discussing treatment goals, exploring alternatives, engaging in shared decision-making, requesting written information, and scheduling follow-up appointments, you actively shape your treatment plan and contribute to your overall well-being.

Navigating Financial Waters: A Comprehensive Guide to Managing Parkinson's Healthcare Costs

Embarking on the journey of living with Parkinson's brings not only physical and emotional challenges but also considerations of the financial aspects of healthcare. In this exploration, we'll delve into the realm of financial considerations, offering insights and strategies to help you explore resources and effectively manage healthcare costs.

UNDERSTANDING THE LANDSCAPE: Financial Implications of Parkinson's
Living with Parkinson's often involves ongoing medical care, medications, and potentially, additional support services. As you navigate these waters, it's crucial to address the financial aspects with the same diligence as other facets of your journey.

Assessing Your Current Financial Situation

Why? Understanding your financial standing is the first step in effective planning.

How: Begin by assessing your current financial situation. Consider your income, savings, and any existing insurance coverage. Identify potential areas of financial strain and determine how your Parkinson's-related expenses may impact your overall budget.

Reviewing Insurance Coverage

Why? Comprehensive insurance coverage can significantly alleviate healthcare costs.

How: Review your existing insurance policies, including health insurance, Medicare, or Medicaid. Understand the coverage details, including co-pays, deductibles, and any limitations related to Parkinson's treatments. If needed, explore supplemental insurance options that may enhance coverage.

Exploring Patient Assistance Programs and Resources

Why? Patient assistance programs offer valuable financial support.

How: Investigate pharmaceutical company programs and nonprofit organizations that provide financial assistance for medications and treatments related to Parkinson's. These programs can offer relief by covering or reducing the cost of prescribed medications and certain medical expenses.

Utilizing Government Assistance Programs

Why? Government programs can offer additional financial support.

How: Explore government assistance programs such as Social Security Disability Insurance (SSDI) or Supplemental Security Income (SSI). These programs can provide financial aid to individuals with disabilities, including those with Parkinson's disease.

Creating a Healthcare Budget

Why? A well-planned budget ensures financial stability amid healthcare expenses.

How: Develop a detailed healthcare budget that includes anticipated medical costs, medication expenses, and any out-of-pocket expenditures. Consider allocating funds for potential emergencies or unexpected healthcare needs. Regularly review and adjust your budget as needed.

Engaging in Open Communication with Healthcare Providers

Why? Transparent communication with healthcare providers can lead to cost-effective solutions.

How: Discuss your financial concerns with your healthcare team. They may be able to suggest generic alternatives, provide samples of medications, or recommend cost-effective treatment options without compromising quality care. Healthcare professionals can be valuable allies in managing costs.

Exploring Financial Assistance for Medical Equipment

Why? Medical equipment costs can be a significant part of Parkinson's care.

How: Investigate programs and organizations that offer financial assistance or discounted rates for medical equipment such as mobility aids or home modifications. Your healthcare team or local Parkinson's support groups may provide recommendations.

Considering Long-Term Care Planning

Why? Long-term care planning provides financial security for the future.

How: Evaluate long-term care options and associated costs. This may include in-home care, assisted living facilities, or nursing homes. Understanding these potential future expenses allows you to plan ahead and make informed decisions.

Researching Tax Deductions and Credits

Why? Tax deductions and credits can provide financial relief.
How: Familiarize yourself with tax deductions and credits applicable to medical expenses. Keep detailed records of healthcare-related costs, including co-pays, travel expenses for medical appointments, and home modifications. Consult with a tax professional to ensure you maximize available benefits.

Seeking Guidance from Financial Advisors

Why? Financial advisors can provide personalized advice.
How: Consult with a financial advisor experienced in healthcare planning. They can help you navigate complex financial considerations, create a comprehensive financial plan, and explore investment strategies to support your long-term healthcare needs.

Addressing the financial aspects of living with Parkinson's requires careful planning, exploration of available resources, and open communication with healthcare providers. By assessing your financial situation, reviewing insurance coverage, exploring assistance programs, creating a healthcare budget, engaging with healthcare providers, researching long-term care options, considering tax benefits, and seeking guidance from financial advisors, you can navigate the financial landscape with confidence and focus on what matters most—your well-being.

Navigating Long-Term Care Options: Planning for Your Future with Informed Choices

As we journey through life, it's essential to consider not only the present but also the future, especially when living with Parkinson's disease. Long-term care planning is a crucial aspect of preparing for the road ahead, ensuring that you have the necessary support and resources to maintain quality of life as your needs evolve.

In this discussion, I'll explore the practicalities of navigating long-term care options, empowering you to make informed choices tailored to your unique circumstances.

Understanding the Need for Long-Term Care

Living with Parkinson's involves a progressive journey, and as symptoms evolve, so do care needs. Long-term care encompasses a range of services designed to support individuals with chronic conditions in maintaining their independence and well-being. Whether you're currently in the early stages of Parkinson's or further along in your journey, planning for long-term care is a proactive step towards ensuring your future comfort and security.

ASSESSING YOUR CARE NEEDS:

The first step in navigating long-term care options is to assess your current and anticipated care needs. Consider the following factors:

- Daily Activities: Evaluate your ability to perform daily tasks independently, such as dressing, bathing, and meal preparation.
- Mobility: Assess your mobility and any assistance you may require for safe movement within your home and community.
- Medication Management: Consider your ability to manage medications effectively and whether you may need assistance with medication reminders or administration.
- Safety: Identify any safety concerns within your home environment and potential modifications or assistance needed to ensure your safety.
- Social and Emotional Support: Reflect on your social network and emotional well-being, recognizing the importance of social engagement and emotional support in maintaining overall well-being.

EXPLORING LONG-TERM CARE OPTIONS

Once you've assessed your care needs, it's time to explore the available long-term care options:

- Home-Based Care: Home care services provide assistance with activities of daily living, medication management, and companionship within the comfort of your own home.
- Assisted Living Facilities: Assisted living facilities offer a supportive environment with assistance available as needed, while still allowing for independence and social engagement.
- Nursing Homes: Nursing homes provide round-the-clock skilled nursing care for individuals with more complex medical needs or those requiring intensive supervision and assistance.
- Memory Care Facilities: Memory care facilities specialize in providing care for individuals with cognitive impairments, such as dementia or Parkinson's-related dementia, offering tailored support and programming.
- Hospice Care: Hospice care focuses on providing comfort and support for individuals with advanced illness, including Parkinson's, with a focus on enhancing quality of life and managing symptoms.

MAKING INFORMED CHOICES

When making decisions about long-term care, it's essential to consider the following factors:

- Personal Preferences: Reflect on your preferences regarding location, amenities, and level of care.
- Financial Considerations: Evaluate the cost of long-term care options and explore available resources, such as insurance coverage, government assistance programs, and personal savings.
- Quality of Care: Research and visit potential care facilities to assess their reputation, staff qualifications, safety measures, and overall quality of care.
- Future Needs: Anticipate how your care needs may change over time and choose a care option that can adapt to your evolving requirements.
- Legal and Advance Care Planning: Ensure that your legal documents, such as advance directives and powers of attorney, are in place to guide medical and financial decisions in the event of incapacity.

ENGAGING WITH YOUR SUPPORT NETWORK

Navigating long-term care options can feel overwhelming, but remember that you don't have to do it alone. Lean on your support network, including family members, friends, healthcare providers, and social workers, for guidance and assistance throughout the decision-making process. Their insights and support can offer valuable perspective and reassurance as you plan for the future.

Planning for long-term care requires careful consideration, research, and proactive decision-making. By assessing your care needs, exploring available options, making informed choices, and engaging with your support network, you can navigate the long-term care landscape with confidence and peace of mind, knowing that you've taken proactive steps to ensure your future comfort and well-being.

CHAPTER 8

Looking Ahead: The Future of Parkinson's Research and Treatment

Exploring the Frontier of Parkinson's Research: A Glimpse into Promising Avenues

As we stand at the frontier of Parkinson's research, the landscape is evolving with exciting prospects that hold the potential to redefine the way we approach and treat this condition. In this exploration, I'll delve into the promising avenues of stem cell therapy, gene therapy, and other advancements that offer hope for the future. This journey of discovery aims to provide you with insights into the cutting-edge developments that may shape the landscape of Parkinson's treatment.

STEM CELL THERAPY: Nurturing Hope at the Cellular Level

Stem cell therapy represents a groundbreaking approach in Parkinson's research, harnessing the regenerative power of stem cells to restore function and repair damaged tissues. Here's a closer look at key aspects of stem cell therapy:

- Understanding Stem Cells: Stem cells possess the remarkable ability to transform into various cell types within the body. Researchers explore how these adaptable cells can be harnessed to replace damaged neurons in the brains of individuals with Parkinson's.

- Dopamine Production: One of the hallmark features of Parkinson's is the loss of dopamine-producing neurons. Stem cell therapy aims to replenish dopamine levels by introducing new, healthy neurons derived from stem cells, potentially alleviating motor symptoms.

- Clinical Trials and Progress: The field of stem cell therapy for Parkinson's is advancing through rigorous clinical trials. Encouraging results have been observed, suggesting that this innovative approach could pave the way for disease-modifying treatments in the future.

GENE THERAPY: Unlocking the Potential within Our DNA
Gene therapy holds the promise of addressing the underlying genetic factors that contribute to Parkinson's disease. This cutting-edge approach involves manipulating genes to modify

or replace faulty genetic material. Key elements of gene therapy include:

- Targeting Genetic Mutations: Researchers are identifying specific genetic mutations associated with Parkinson's and exploring ways to correct or replace these faulty genes. This personalized approach aims to address the root causes of the disease.
- Optimizing Neurotransmitter Levels: Gene therapy also seeks to regulate neurotransmitter levels, including dopamine, by introducing genes that enhance their production or release. This approach may offer a more precise and sustainable method of symptom management.
- Advancements in Viral Vectors: Delivering therapeutic genes into the brain requires specialized carriers called viral vectors. Ongoing advancements in viral vector technology enhance the precision and safety of gene therapy applications for Parkinson's.

OTHER ADVANCEMENTS IN PARKINSON'S RESEARCH: A Holistic Approach

Beyond stem cell and gene therapies, researchers are exploring a spectrum of advancements that take a holistic approach to Parkinson's management:

- Neuroprotective Strategies: Investigating compounds and interventions that can protect existing neurons from degeneration is a key focus. This may include antioxidants, anti-inflammatory agents, and other neuroprotective approaches.
- Innovations in Deep Brain Stimulation (DBS): Refinements in DBS techniques continue to enhance its effectiveness in managing motor symptoms. Researchers are exploring novel electrode placements, stimulation patterns, and adaptive technologies to optimize outcomes.
- Biochemical Pathways and Drug Development: Understanding the intricate biochemical pathways involved in Parkinson's pathology is guiding the development of targeted medications. Novel drugs aim to modulate these pathways for more precise and effective symptom management.
- Advances in Wearable Technology: Wearable devices equipped with sensors and artificial intelligence are being explored to monitor and analyze subtle changes in

motor function. This technology offers real-time data that can inform personalized treatment plans.

As we navigate the evolving landscape of Parkinson's research, it's important to recognize the collaborative effort involving scientists, healthcare professionals, individuals living with Parkinson's, and their support networks. Each advancement, each discovery, brings us closer to a future where the impact of Parkinson's can be mitigated, if not halted.

While these promising avenues are not yet standard treatments, they offer a beacon of hope and a testament to the dedication of the scientific community. The journey continues, and with it, the anticipation of a brighter tomorrow for those affected by Parkinson's.

Personalized Medicine in Parkinson's: Tailoring Hope to Your Unique Journey

As we delve into the realm of Parkinson's research, one of the most promising frontiers is personalized medicine—a groundbreaking approach that seeks to tailor treatment to the individual needs of each person living with Parkinson's. This journey of exploration unfolds the potential of personalized medicine, offering a glimpse into how this innovative approach could revolutionize the landscape of Parkinson's care, providing hope that is distinctly crafted for you.

UNDERSTANDING PERSONALIZED MEDICINE: A Customized Path to Well-Being

Personalized medicine, also known as precision medicine, recognizes that every person's experience with Parkinson's is unique. It embraces the idea that a one-size-fits-all approach may not be the most effective, considering the diverse range of symptoms, genetic factors, and lifestyle variations among individuals.

Key Elements of Personalized Medicine:

- Genetic Profiling: One of the cornerstones of personalized medicine is the in-depth analysis of an individual's genetic makeup. By understanding specific genetic variations associated with Parkinson's, healthcare providers can tailor interventions to address the root causes at a molecular level.
- Biomarker Identification: Personalized medicine also relies on identifying biomarkers—indicators in the body that reflect the presence or progression of the disease. These biomarkers guide healthcare

professionals in monitoring the effectiveness of treatments and adjusting them as needed.

- Lifestyle and Environmental Factors: Beyond genetics, personalized medicine considers lifestyle and environmental factors that influence Parkinson's progression. These may include diet, exercise, exposure to toxins, and other elements that contribute to an individual's overall health.

THE Step-by-Step JOURNEY OF PERSONALIZED MEDICINE:

Comprehensive Assessment:

Why: The first step involves a comprehensive assessment of your medical history, symptoms, and genetic profile.

How: Engage with your healthcare team in open and transparent communication. Share your experiences, concerns, and any relevant family medical history. This forms the foundation for a personalized approach.

Genetic Profiling:

Why: Understanding your genetic predisposition is crucial for tailoring interventions.

How: Undergo genetic testing to identify specific genetic variations associated with Parkinson's. This information enables healthcare providers to create a targeted plan that addresses the unique aspects of your condition.

Biomarker Identification:

Why: Biomarkers provide real-time insights into disease progression and treatment effectiveness.

How: Your healthcare team may conduct tests, such as imaging scans or blood tests, to identify biomarkers. Regular monitoring of these biomarkers informs adjustments to your treatment plan, ensuring it remains aligned with your evolving needs.

Lifestyle and Environmental Analysis:

Why: Lifestyle and environmental factors significantly impact Parkinson's.

How: Collaborate with your healthcare team to assess aspects like diet, exercise, and exposure to potential environmental triggers. Make informed choices to optimize your lifestyle for better overall well-being.

Tailored Treatment Plan:

Why: Personalized medicine enables the creation of a treatment plan uniquely suited to your condition.

How: Based on the comprehensive assessment, genetic profiling, and biomarker identification, your healthcare team will craft a personalized treatment plan. This may include targeted medications, therapies, and lifestyle recommendations tailored to address your specific challenges.

Continuous Monitoring and Adjustment:
Why: Parkinson's is dynamic, and treatment plans need to evolve accordingly.
How: Regular follow-ups with your healthcare team allow for continuous monitoring of your condition. Biomarkers and ongoing assessments guide adjustments to your treatment plan, ensuring it remains responsive to your changing needs.

Embracing personalized medicine is a collaborative effort between you and your healthcare team. Active participation, open communication, and a commitment to making informed lifestyle choices empower you to take an active role in your personalized treatment journey.

As we explore the potential of personalized medicine in Parkinson's, it becomes clear that hope is not a generic concept but a uniquely crafted path tailored to your individual journey. By embracing personalized medicine, we step into a future where the power of precision transforms the landscape of Parkinson's care, offering new possibilities for a life lived to the fullest.

CHAPTER 9

A Final Note: Living Beyond Limitations

Recap and Empowering Messages: Navigating Parkinson's with Resilience

As we reflect on our discussions, let's distill the essence into key takeaways that empower you to navigate the journey of Parkinson's with resilience, hope, and a proactive spirit. This recap is a reminder that, despite the challenges, there are tools, insights, and a supportive community to guide you towards a fulfilling life beyond the tremors.

1. Shifting the Narrative: Beyond Tremors
Key Takeaway: Parkinson's is more than tremors. Embrace a holistic understanding of the condition, acknowledging both motor and non-motor aspects.

2. Dispelling Myths and Fostering Hope

Key Takeaway: Separate fact from fiction. Early intervention is powerful, and advancements in research offer hope for a brighter future.

3. Building Your Wellness Arsenal: Traditional Therapies
Key Takeaway: Understand the medication landscape, explore surgical interventions like DBS, and embrace physical and occupational therapies for a comprehensive approach to well-being.

4. Exploring Complementary and Alternative Therapies
Key Takeaway: Complement traditional therapies with mind-body approaches, nutritional considerations, and complementary therapies to enhance overall health.

5. The Power of Your Network: Navigating Support Systems
Key Takeaway: Build a robust support team, connect with patient advocacy groups, communicate effectively, and address emotional challenges with resilience.

6. Living Well, Not Just Managing
Key Takeaway: Set realistic goals, adapt hobbies, travel thoughtfully, and maintain intimate relationships to redefine your quality of life.

7. Taking Charge of Your Healthcare: Advocacy and Exploration

Key Takeaway: Be an active participant in your healthcare journey. Engage in clinical trials, manage financial considerations, and plan for the future with informed choices.

8. Looking Ahead: Future of Parkinson's Research and Treatment

Key Takeaway: Stay informed about promising research avenues, personalized medicine, and the importance of continued support for ongoing advancements.

9. Living Beyond Limitations: A Final Note

Key Takeaway: Recap the journey with an emphasis on empowerment. You have the tools, support, and resilience to live beyond limitations, embracing a fulfilling life with Parkinson's.

Empowering Message: A Call to Action

As you absorb these key takeaways, remember that Parkinson's is a chapter in your life, not the entire story. Your journey is unique, filled with possibilities, triumphs, and the strength to overcome challenges. Embrace the support around you, stay informed, and cultivate a mindset that sees beyond the diagnosis. You are not defined by Parkinson's; rather, it's an aspect of your life that you can navigate with grace and determination.

Conclusion: Embracing a Future of Resilience and Possibility

As we conclude this journey together, I want to extend my deepest appreciation for embarking on this exploration of Parkinson's with me. This book has been a labor of love, a testament to the strength, resilience, and boundless potential that reside within each person facing the challenges of Parkinson's disease.

In these pages, we've traversed a landscape of understanding, dispelling myths, and embracing a comprehensive approach to well-being. It's not just a book; it's a conversation about living beyond the tremors, about finding unexpected tools, and about thriving despite the challenges that Parkinson's may bring.

As you close these pages, I encourage you to carry forward the spirit of empowerment, the knowledge gained, and the stories of resilience. Remember, you are not alone on this journey.

The Parkinson's community is a tapestry of shared experiences, support, and collective strength.

In the face of Parkinson's, we find not only a diagnosis but an opportunity—an opportunity to redefine what it means to live a fulfilling life. It's about setting realistic goals, celebrating victories, and adapting with grace. You are not defined by Parkinson's; you are defined by your resilience, your courage, and your ability to navigate a path forward.

As you step beyond the pages of this book, know that the journey continues. Stay engaged with your healthcare team, connect with the Parkinson's community, and be an advocate for your well-being. The unexpected tools you've discovered are now in your hands, ready to shape a future filled with resilience and possibility.

Thank you for allowing me to be a part of your journey. May the chapters ahead be filled with hope, strength, and the unwavering belief in the potential for a fulfilling life with Parkinson's.

Onward,

Linda J. Scott.